The Special Senses

George J. McKenzie BA RGN RMN RNT
Lecturer in Nursing Studies,
Dundee College of Technology, Dundee

Hector Bryson Chawla MB ChB(St And) DO(Lond)
DRCOG(Lond) FRCS(Edin)
Consultant Ophthalmic Surgeon, Royal Infirmary, Edinburgh;
Examiner, Royal College of Surgeons, Edinburgh and
Royal College of Physicians and Surgeons, Glasgow

David Gordon BSc MB FRCS
Senior Registrar, Department of Otolaryngology,
Ninewells Hospital, Dundee

SECOND EDITION

CHURCHILL LIVINGSTONE
EDINBURGH LONDON MELBOURNE AND NEW YORK 1986

CHURCHILL LIVINGSTONE
Medical Division of Longman Group Limited

Distributed in the United States of America by Churchill
Livingstone Inc., 1560 Broadway, New York, N.Y. 10036,
and by associated companies, branches and representatives
throughout the world.

First edition 1976
Second edition 1986

ISBN 0-443-03081-2

British Library Cataloguing in Publication Data
McKenzie, George J.
    The special senses. — 2nd ed.
    1. Ophthalmic nursing   2. Otolarynogological
nursing
    I. Title   II. Chawla, Hector Bryson   III. Gordon,
David   IV. Casey, T. A.
    617'.51'0024613   RE88

Produced by Longman Singapore Publishers (Pte) Ltd.
Printed in Singapore

Preface

The treatment of disorders affecting the special senses has been revolutionised over the past two to three decades. The advent of the operating microscope, new anaesthetic techniques, new suture materials and new drugs has brought about many changes in the way disorders are treated and hence in the way patients are nursed.

This second edition has been extensively rewritten to take account of changes in treatment and nursing care. It has been assumed that the reader will already have mastered fundamental nursing skills so these have not been elaborated on to any extent. The basic needs of an individual with a disorder affecting the special senses is the same as for any other person. Where vision and/or hearing are impaired the patient may often require some additional assistance with the activities of daily living. Nursing care needs to be adapted in a way which will enable the patient to remain as independent as possible. A person newly deaf or blind requires a great deal of support and encouragement whilst he is adapting to his sudden loss. Many of the frustrations endured by the deaf or blind are made worse by the way other people respond to them. Given also that many of these people are elderly, nursing the person with loss of hearing or vision is a challenging and rewarding activity.

This small book is not intended as a definitive nursing/surgical/medical text, but is written with the student nurse in mind so that her experience in the otorhinolaryngology or ophthalmology ward may be made more interesting by her understanding of the conditions afflicting her patients. It should also be of interest to nurses in other clinical areas and in the community who will inevitably, at some stage, encounter patients with ear, nose and throat or eye problems or with impaired hearing or vision.

Many completely new illustrations have been added. We are grateful to A. Chilman and M. Thomas for the use of a few illustrations from *Understanding Nursing Care*, and in addition acknowledge the use of many of the illustrations from H. Chawla's *Essential Ophthalmology*. Both books are published by Churchill Livingstone, Edinburgh.

The authors are grateful to colleagues and the publishers for all their help and guidance during the production of this new edition.

Dundee, 1986   G. J. McK.
                                                          H. C.
                                                          D. G.

Contents

Introduction
Admission to hospital

On being admitted to hospital, most patients will be aware of the diagnosis and the reasons for admission. For most people, submitting themselves to surgery will not have been an easy decision. Most patients will have had various tests and investigations and/or treatment as out-patients, and so will have had some preparation for their stay in hospital. In spite of this, few people relish the thought of coming into hospital, especially for surgery, and are inevitably anxious about what is going to happen to them. Also, when we remember how much importance we attach to our sight and hearing, operations and treatment for eye and ear conditions give rise to perhaps more anxiety than most operations. After all, we only have to close our eyes to get some idea of what it is like to be blind; though it is more difficult to imagine what it must be like to be deaf. Many patients will, of course, have had experience in hospital on previous occasions for the treatment of eye and ear disorders. This may or may not lessen their fears; much depends on what it is hoped the latest treatment proposed will achieve. Not all patients coming into the ophthalmic and otorhinolaryngology wards are elective admissions. Emergency admissions to both these specialised units are very common, mostly as a result of accidents. Special aspects in the care of emergency admissions will be discussed when the specific condition is dealt with. Suffice it to say that most, if not all, of what follows regarding elective admissions applies equally well to emergency admissions also.

Medical history and diagnosis

The doctor will conduct a detailed medical examination on admission. This enables the doctor to take a history of the present illness and to identify what the patient's chief complaint is. The patient's past history and any concurrent illness or disability is noted. This is important as it is all too easy to neglect concurrent illnesses such as heart disease, diabetes etc. Coming into hospital upsets the individual's routine, and disorders such as diabetes mellitus can all too easily become unstable and pose an additional risk. The doctor may not be able to make a final diagnosis on admission and may wish various further investigations to be made to make certain.

Nursing history

The nursing history and assessment of the patient differs from the medical history in that it is patient-problem centred. It is more concerned with the effects of the medical diagnosis on the patient and his perspective of his illness. In taking the nursing history, the nurse hopes to elicit the patient's needs and personal priorities. The nurse is primarily concerned with the preservation of bodily functions and the prevention of complications which may arise as a result of his medical/surgical treatment, enforced rest or other factors which may be obstacles in the way of his optimum recovery. The nursing history is a means of assessing the patients' total health needs—not just his present needs but also his future needs. Only after systematic assessment and analysis of the findings can an individualised nursing care plan be devised. Failure to properly identify the patient's needs accurately will mean that both actual and potential problems/needs may be missed. It is not possible to discuss interview techniques and detailed nursing history formats in a book of this size, but this information is widely available in any of the better foundation nursing books; see Further Reading on page 204.

Pre-operative tests and investigations

Many pre-operative tests will be done before admission, but many are conducted after admission and others repeated. The pre-operative tests fall into two categories. In the first category are those relating specifically to the ENT or eye disorder, e.g. hearing tests, electro-nystagmography, caloric studies and special X-rays of the head and neck. Eye investigations include tests for visual acuity, visual field tests, measurements of intra-ocular pressure and the patency of the tear ducts.

Secondly, there are tests which establish the general fitness of the patient and confirm the diagnosis if it has not been clearly established. These are, of course, essential before anaesthesia and surgery. Many tests in both eye and ENT wards are done by the doctors or by other specially trained paramedical staff. Some investigations, however, are essentially nursing functions. These include urinalysis to test for sugar, protein, etc. and base line recordings of temperature pulse and blood pressure. The latter are vital for post-operation comparisons. Most patients will have blood tests such as haemoglobin, blood urea and electrolytes measured. Some will also require a chest X-ray, electrocardiogram and pulmonary function tests. It is most important that the patient is kept informed of why particular tests are necessary and of the results. This will help to relieve anxiety and make the individual feel that he is still in control of events, if only just.

Informed consent

The doctor will explain the nature of any treatment or surgery proposed and get the patient to sign a consent form agreeing to any operation. It is important that the patient should have a good understanding of the treatment proposed, the expected outcome and possible complications. The doctor will also explain any alterative treatment or likely outcome if no treatment is agreed to. Only by doing this can the patient participate realistically in decisions regarding the treatment of his disorder. Not all treatments will be successful and hoped for improvements may not be immediately apparent. For example, hearing may not be obviously better on first removal of bandages, nor may vision be anything like perfect on removal of eyepads. Nurses need to be conversant with these facts, and many more, about eye and ENT disorders and their treatments so that they can reassure without causing alarm or raising false hopes.

Good pre-operative instruction helps to avoid such disappointments. Should the nurse discover that the patient does not fully understand the nature of his problem and the treatment proposed, she should be able to explain the situation to the patient. She should also inform the doctor who may also want to clarify things for the patient, especially in matters relating to prognosis or if the nurse is not completely sure of the disorder and its therapy herself.

If the patient has a known or suspected cancer the consultant must also decide how much the patient should be told. He should inform the nurses of his decision. This is very necessary if the patient is going to get consistent information from all concerned. Wrong information can lead to misunderstandings and increased anxiety. The patient's relatives may not wish the patient to know the truth. Attitudes vary considerably and every patient must be assessed individually. There is no room for blanket decisions in these circumstances. The majority of patients will be told of the diagnosis. This makes explanation of treatments such as radiotherapy, radical surgery and chemotherapy easier, and avoids the situation where everyone knows or thinks he knows but nobody talks about it—a conspiracy of silence!

Preparation for surgery

It is the nurse's responsibility to finally prepare the patient for his operation and to familiarise him with the post-operation events he may experience. Good pre-operative care leads to fewer complications. Patients require less analgesia, are more easily mobilised and can be discharged earlier. The nurse must always bear in mind the strangeness of the surgical experience to the patient. To him it is a novel and terrifying ordeal and is usually undertaken with a good degree of foreboding. The patient wants to know what is to happen and how he can help. Preferably one nurse should be responsible for preparing the patient for surgery. He should be told which part of the ward he will be returning to so that he does not wake up in completely strange surroundings. If he is going to an intensive care unit or some other ward he should be informed of this and given reasons. Patients also need to be told of any wounds they may have, including information about drains or packs which may be in situ. For example, a patient recovering from anaesthesia with bilateral nose packs may find it difficult to breathe and hence struggle and remove packs which could lead to unnecessary complications. In some of the more major operations, e.g. laryngectomy, intravenous infusions and naso-gastric tubes will be required as well as humidification for the tracheostomy. A brief explanation should be given so that the patient is not completely overwhelmed by it all on recovery from anaesthesia. Similarly, following major eye surgery the eyes may be padded for a day or two and this can be very alarming, especially for the patient who has previously been able to see. Good pre-operative instructions make it easier for the patient to cope post-operatively. In short, the patient has to learn new skills to enable him to deal with what is, after all, a new and more than likely frightening experience.

Pain

It is pain patients fear most about surgery and few operations are painless. It is best to tell the patient he will experience pain but that this will be relieved by pain-relieving drugs, and that these will be given regularly so that pain is kept to a minimum. It is important to create an atmosphere of trust and understanding.

Anaesthetist's visit

The anaesthetist will visit the patient before the operation to assess his general condition, get to know the patient a little and prescribe a premedication. This visit is reassuring for the patient, making him feel that the whole team care about him as an individual.

Multidisciplinary team

Before more major surgery (e.g. laryngectomy) the physiotherapist will also visit the patient to give instructions on deep breathing and expectoration. It is best if the patient learns this before the surgery as it makes it easier for him afterwards. Other specialists, such as speech therapists, audiologists and dietitians, will be consulted as required. Ear, nose and throat surgery is very much a team effort.

The exact requirements for each operation will become apparent as you read about the specific conditions and treatments throughout the book.

For details of general pre-operative care and anaesthesia the nurse should refer to a foundation nursing textbook (see p. 204).

Post-operative care

On completion of the operation, the care of the patient will be taken over by the recovery room staff. Recovery time from the anaesthetic will usually be quite short. However, attention to airways and vital signs is obligatory. Once the patient has recovered from the anaesthetic and the anaesthetist is satisfied that his condition is stable, arrangements will be made for the patient's return to the ward. If possible, the nurse who prepared the patient and took him to the theatre should also collect him from the theatre. This nurse is responsible for the safe transport of the patient back to the ward area. She should collect all notes, charts and X-rays and receive a report on the patient's condition, the type of operation performed and any special post-operative instructions. The patient is then transported back to the ward or intensive care area which will have been previously prepared for his return. His positioning in bed will be determined by the nature of the operation, drains, etc. As soon as the patient is positioned safely, the airway, wounds, drains, etc. should be checked and his vital signs recorded. Serial recordings of T.P.R. and B/P are established and a fluid balance chart is commenced if necessary. What happens next depends on the nature of the operation.

Section I

The ear, nose and throat

Caring for patients with ear, nose and throat diseases is a specialist field of nursing and involves the care of all age groups. Disorders of the ear, nose and throat are very common. Who has not at some time suffered a sore throat or a nose bleed? However, the range of ear, nose and throat disorders are not confined to sore throats and nose bleeds, as you will discover when you read this book. The scope of ear, nose and throat surgery ranges from major operations, such as total laryngectomy for cancer, to microscopic reconstruction of the auditory ossicles.

Infections of the upper respiratory tract are amongst the most common to afflict man. Most infections are self-limiting and, after causing the individual a few days discomfort, they resolve naturally and are quickly forgotten about. Some infections, however, do not resolve completely and become chronic. Even today, in spite of all the antibiotics and other treatments available, they can still cause serious problems. For example, chronic middle ear infections can destroy the auditory ossicles and seriously impair hearing. Infection may even penetrate through the skull and result in a cerebral abscess. Similarly, acute ethmoidal sinusitis can press on the optic nerve and orbit and impair vision.

Injuries to the head and neck are also very common. In many cases, damage will occur to either the ear, nose or throat. Injuries range from fractures of the nose and larynx, to laceration of the tympanic membrane from blast injuries.

Tumours, whilst not very common, can have a devastating effect. Being suddenly without a voice and our main means of communication from an acute laryngitis is bad enough. Being permanently deprived of a voice because of the need for a laryngectomy is for most of us too difficult to comprehend.

Lastly, we should not forget the various congenital defects, the most serious being deafness. Significant numbers of children are born deaf each year. At present, surgery has perhaps not a lot to offer this group but certainly has more to offer those with acquired deafness, especially the conductive type. Sensorineural deafness is not so amenable to surgery but research continues all the while and, with the advent of the microchip and other sophisticated electronics, help may one day be available for this group also. From this brief introduction it can be seen that the scope of ear, nose and throat nursing involves caring for a patient with a wide range of disorders.

The majority of patients with ear, nose and throat disorders are treated by their own doctor and administer their own medication. Many, however, do require hospital treatment. Patients admitted for ear, nose and throat surgery are seldom detained long: some for only a day or two and most for no more than two weeks. This can make it difficult to get to know the patients very well. This, however, is no excuse for nurses not taking time to assess the patient's needs. Because the patient is only in hospital for a short period and may have to continue his treatment at home, an ability to win the patient's co-operation and, hence, compliance in self-care is essential. The nurse's level of knowledge and mastery of skills instills confidence in her patients which help them to achieve optimal recovery, or adaptation to their handicap.

One
The ear

Applied anatomy and physiology

The ear is divided anatomically into outer, middle and inner parts
(Fig. 1.1). The pinna is a cartilaginous structure covered by perichondrium and skin which are tightly bound to it. The external
auditory canal is about one inch in length. Its skeleton is cartilaginous in its outer third and bony in the inner two thirds. The lining
skin of the outer third is hair-bearing and also contains the cerum-

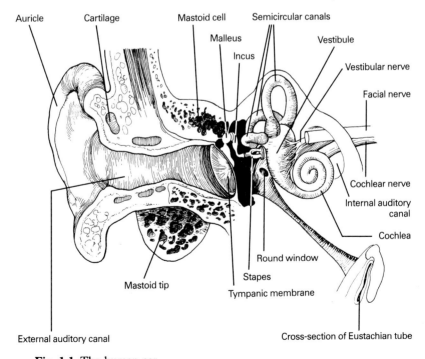

Fig. 1.1 The human ear

inous glands which are responsible for wax secretion, whilst that of the inner two thirds is thin and very sensitive to the touch.

The tympanic membrane consists of three layers: an outer squamous epithelium, a middle fibrous layer and an inner lining mucous membrane. It is divided into the larger pars tensa inferiorly, while the upper part of the membrane has no fibrous layer and is called the pars flaccida. The healthy drum is a bright silver colour and is seen to reflect light back to the examining eye. The handle, short process and lateral process of the malleus are landmarks which can be seen on it (Fig. 1.2).

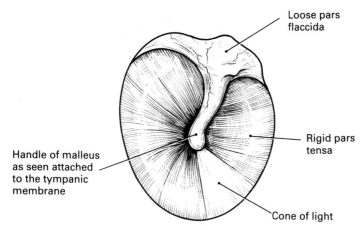

Loose pars flaccida

Rigid pars tensa

Handle of malleus as seen attached to the tympanic membrane

Cone of light

Fig. 1.2 A normal tympanic membrane as viewed down the external auditory canal.

The middle ear or tympanic cavity lies behind the tympanic membrane (Fig. 1.3). The middle ear cavity is ventilated by way of the Eustachian tube. The Eustachian tube extends from the middle ear cavity to the nasopharynx (Fig. 1.1). The upper part of the cavity, above the tympanic membrane, is the attic region which is connected to the mastoid antrum via a short aditus. The antrum in turn connects with multiple mastoid air cells. It can, therefore, be seen that the most distant mastoid cell has a direct connection with the nasopharynx via an air-filled system.

The anatomical relationships of the middle ear and mastoid system are important. The roof or tegmen of the tympanic cavity separates it from the temporal lobe of the brain. The facial nerve runs within a bony canal on its medial and posterior wall where it gives off the chorda tympani nerve, which runs through the cavity. It supplies taste to the anterior two thirds of the tongue and may

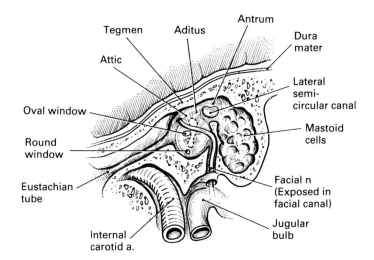

Fig. 1.3 The tympanic cavity.

be damaged during middle ear surgery. Lying medial to the middle ear are the inner ear structures. The cerebellum and lateral venous sinus lie closely related to the mastoid air cells.

As a result of these close relationships, infection of the middle ear, if allowed to spread, may cause serious complications. Likewise, fractures of the skull in this area may damage several important structures.

The air-containing middle ear cavity encloses three ossicles (Fig. 1.4). The head of the malleus forms a joint with the body of the incus in the attic. The long process of the incus in turn runs down to connect with the head of the stapes. This last ossicle, shaped like a stirrup, lies with its footplate in the oval window which opens into the inner ear. A second opening called the round window can also be seen just inferior to the oval window.

The anatomy of the inner ear is complex (Fig. 1.5). It accommodates both the cochlear and vestibular systems which serve hearing the balance respectively. The system consists of an inner membranous labyrinth, whose odd shape can be seen in the diagram. This structure is filled with endolymphatic fluid and in turn is completely surrounded by perilymphatic fluid, which separates it from a similarly shaped bony labyrinth.

The anterior part of the system is the cochlea. This is spiral in shape and when seen in cross section the relationship between the membranous and bony labyrinths becomes a little clearer (Figs. 1.6a and b). Within the membranous compartment lies the organ

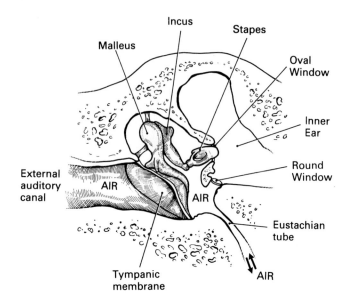

Fig. 1.4 Normal ear: air pressure on tympanic membrane equal on both sides.

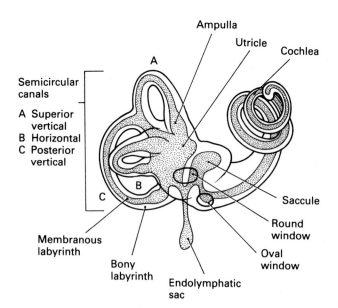

Fig. 1.5 Inner ear structure.

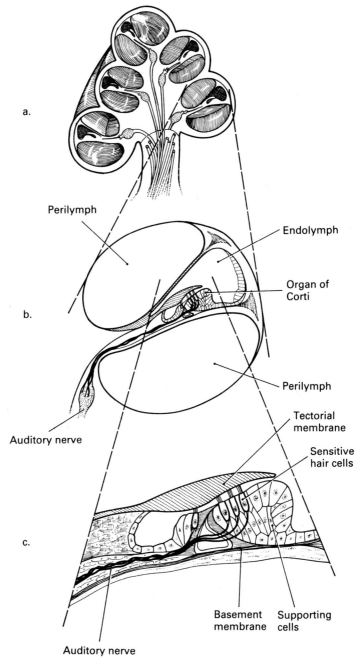

a.

b.

c.

Perilymph

Endolymph

Organ of
Corti

Perilymph

Tectorial
membrane

Sensitive
hair cells

Auditory nerve

Basement   Supporting
membrane   cells

Auditory nerve

Fig. 1.6 (a) Cross section of the cochlea. (b) Relationship between the
bony and membranous labyrinth. (c) Organ of Corti.

of Corti (Fig. 1.6c), bathed in endolymph. Sound waves, transmitted through the oval window, travel along the fluid compartments of the cochlea and in so doing distort the basilar lamina which supports the organ, whose hair cells are embedded and fixed into the reticular lamina.

It is the distortion of the hair projections which converts the sound waves into impulses which are transmitted from the Organ of Corti along the 8th nerve to the brain stem and cortex.

The posterior part of the inner ear is formed by the semicircular canals (Fig. 1.5) which are responsible for normal balance. The utricle and saccule contain sensory organs which respond to accelerative forces. This close relationship of middle and inner ear structures is significant for several reasons. As already mentioned, spread of infection may occur. Many middle ear conditions may be associated with disorders of balance, and great care must be taken during microsurgery of the tympanic cavity to avoid disturbance of the labyrinthine structures. In addition, any fluid which is introduced into the ear must be warmed sufficiently to prevent the development of convection currents in the fluid of the semicircular canals. This avoids the onset of vertigo which is very unpleasant and distressing.

Conditions affecting the external canal

Foreign bodies

Many people, but especially small children and the mentally handicapped, insert foreign objects into their ears. Removal may appear to be temptingly easy. However, the risk of damage to the external canal skin or tympanic membrane is high in a struggling toddler who resents any interference. More often than not, general anaesthesia is required for safe removal, although some objects may be cleared by gentle syringing.

Otitis externa

Diffuse inflammation of the skin of the external canal is a surprisingly common and distressing condition. Infection may be introduced by patients who traumatise the skin with the screwed-up corner of a towel or by scratching the ear. A vicious circle of itching and scratching is set up which allows the condition to continue. The condition is characterised by pain (especially if the infection is fungal), itch and discharge. The discharge may be copious (in some reactions); it is usually watery, later becoming purulent. Spread of the infection to the pinna can produce a marked cellulitis which causes systematic upset and pyrexia. The patient feels toxic and generally unwell. The infection is usually caused by a mixture of micro-organisms. A sample of the discharge should be sent on a swab to the bacteriology department for culture and sensitivity of the offending organism.

Treatment and nursing care

Thorough aural toilet is the mainstay of treatment and removal of all infective debris should be achieved by gentle mopping out of the external canal. A Jobson-Horne probe with fluffed cotton wool on the tip is ideal for this. The patient should be seated comfortably and have the procedure carefully explained to him. A good light is essential. Ribbon gauze soaked in a topical antibiotic and steroid preparation can then be inserted and renewed as necessary until the skin settles. Alternatively, preparations in common use are 8% aluminium acetate or ichthammol glycerine. If the condition is extensive, some patients may require hospital admission for treatment with systemic antibiotics, adequate analgesia and bedrest. Care should be taken to prevent infection spreading. Scrupulous hygiene and the careful disposal of contaminated clothing, dressing, etc., are essential. Isolation in a side room will help to prevent the spread of infection and give the patient peace and quiet whilst he is febrile.

Patients should be discouraged from scratching the ears and should prevent water from entering the external canal. Recurrence of the condition is common. The urge to scratch an itching ear proves too difficult to resist for many patients! In some patients, seborrhoeic dermatitis may be a contributing factor and this should be treated with an appropriate medicated shampoo. The old adage not to insert anything larger than your elbow into your ear is worth remembering!

Furunculosis

Furunculosis is an infection of the hair follicles. Occasionally, the hair follicles in the outer third of the auditory canal become infected. The infecting organism is usually a staphylococcus. The main symptom is severe pain with marked tenderness if the pinna is moved. Gentle insertion of an ichthammol and glycerine wick, together with an analgesic, will provide relief from pain, and an antibiotic suitable for staphylococcal infection is the treatment of choice. A well-protected hot water bottle held over the ear may also help to relieve pain and speed up the resolution of the inflammation.

Once the furuncle starts discharging and is draining freely, the external canal should be kept clean by regular aural toilet. The patient's urine should be tested for sugar to exclude diabetes mellitus. Infections of this sort are common in untreated diabetics.

Ear trauma

Injuries to the head and neck are common. Many cases of physical assault and road traffic accidents present daily to Casualty Departments. The structures of the ear, whilst relatively well protected, are delicate and easily damaged, producing severe handicaps.

Trauma to the external ear

A blow to the pinna may cause a haematoma to develop between the cartilage and perichondrium. Drainage of the blood clot must be carried out to prevent it becoming organised with the development of a 'cauliflower' ear, a deformity commonly seen in boxers. Secondary infection of the haematoma results in a perichondritis which will destroy the cartilage of the pinna. The avoidance of perichondritis is also important if the pinna is lacerated. Thorough wound toilet and careful suturing will avoid this complication.

Disorders of the tympanic membrane and the middle ear

Tympanic membrane rupture

A blow to the side of the head with the flat of the hand may seal off the external canal and raise the pressure within it to a level sufficient to rupture the tympanic membrane. Rupture may also arise if, during ear syringing, the full force of the jet of water is directed at the tympanic membrane.

Such injuries produce severe pain and bleeding from the ear. Most of these traumatic perforations will heal spontaneously, provided secondary infection does not develop. It is, therefore, important to recognise such injuries. The patient is advised to keep water out of the ear as with other types of perforation. Damage to the ossicular chain may have occurred at the same time and may explain the persistent deafness after complete healing of the perforation. In many such cases, it will be possible to reconstruct the ossicular chain and, therefore, restore hearing.

Blast injuries to the ear

Explosions result in a very rapid rise in atmospheric pressure which is followed by a period of negative pressure. Blast injuries may cause severe damage to the ear. The positive phase may perforate the tympanic membrane and dislocate the ossicular chain. In addition, severe inner ear damage may also occur.

Barotrauma

During the normal activities of life, the Eustachian tube is well able to maintain the pressure within the middle ear to that of the atmosphere. There are, however, circumstances in which negative pressure may develop: descending from high altitudes whilst flying and in descent whilst diving under water. If pressure equalisation by the Eustachian tube is not efficient, then persistence of the negative pressure produces retraction of the tympanic membrane and the development of pain in the middle ear. Very rapid pressure changes may rupture the tympanic membrane.

The symptoms may be no more than a feeling of 'stuffiness' or 'fullness' in the ear, and a marked deafness. Discomfort and pain may, however, be severe. Poor Eustachian tubal function predisposes to the condition, and for this reason it is unwise for people to fly if they are suffering from an upper respiratory infection. Likewise, divers should not participate in deep water descents if they have a cold.

Serous otitis media

This condition is a common cause of deafness in children. The exact cause is not known. The condition is not well named because it is not a true inflammatory disorder of the middle ear. The fluid which accummulates in the middle ear is often serous but may be thick and viscous, giving rise to its alternative description, namely, 'glue ear'. Normally, the middle ear cavity is air containing. Air enters the cavity via the Eustachian tube. If air is prevented from entering the middle ear cavity by failure of normal tubal function, pressure within the cavity, instead of being equal to atmospheric pressure, becomes negative. This vacuum effect causes the tympanic membrane to become retracted and, in addition, fluid collects within the middle ear (Fig. 1.7a and b). It is this collection of fluid which gives rise to serous otitis media (SOM).

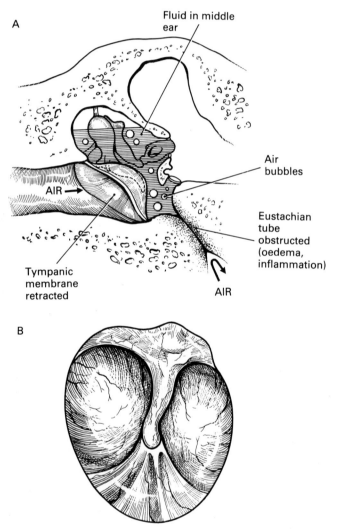

Fig. 1.7 (a) Secretory otitis media (b) Appearance of eardrum in secretory otitis. The negative pressure causes retraction of the tympanic membrane.

Eustachian tubal dysfunction

Eustachian tubal dysfunction may arise for several reasons:

(a) *Upper respiratory infection*, usually viral in origin, is particularly common in children. Involvement of the Eustachian tube results in oedema of the tubal mucosa. The adenoid pad may also enlarge. Both factors will tend to reduce tubal efficiency.

(b) *Cleft palate*. Children with this disorder have poor function of the muscles of the soft palate as a result. Failure to open the Eustachian tube during swallowing leaves these children particularly vulnerable to SOM.

(c) *Tumours of the nasopharynx* may involve the lower end of the tube.

Both tympanic membrane retraction and fluid accumulation will interfere with normal sound transmission. In school-age children, the complaint of deafness is first noticed by the child's mother. It is worth emphasising that such a complaint should always be fully investigated since mothers (in this instance at least) are usually proved correct. In most cases, the deafness is associated with a 'cold' or other respiratory infection.

Treatment

The majority of children will recover spontaneously. However, more active treatment may be required.

(a) *Nasal decongestant drops*, e.g. 0.5% Ephedrine, will reduce nasal oedema and encourage normal Eustachian function. Carbocysteine (Mucodyne) is said to reduce the viscosity of the fluid and may hasten resolution. It is taken orally. If a child is old enough to perform the Valsalva manoeuvre, this is of help in aerating the middle ear.

(b) *Surgical measures* may be required for resistant cases. Drainage of the fluid can be achieved under general anaesthesia by incising the tympanic membrane in the operation of myringotomy (Fig. 1.8). A ventilation tube, called a grommet, is then inserted (Fig. 1.9). This effectively acts as an artificial Eustachian tube and ensures normal middle ear aeration. While grommets remain in place, care should be taken to ensure that no water gets into the

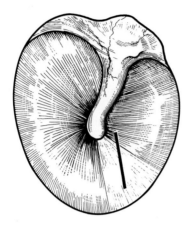

Fig. 1.8 Myringotomy incision.

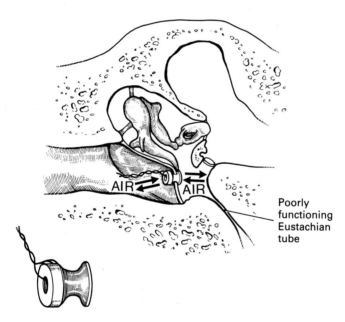

Poorly
functioning
Eustachian
tube

Fig. 1.9 Grommet inserted in the tympanic membrane.

ear during hair washing. Swimming should be forbidden. In general, the grommet falls out of the tympanic membrane in about six months and is extruded from the external canal, usually embedded in wax.

Acute otitis media

Acute bacterial infection of the middle ear is common in childhood and is a distressing condition for both patient and parent. The Eustachian tube provides an easy pathway for the spread of infection to the middle ear cavity. The common cold, sinusitis or infection of the tonsils and adenoids may, therefore, be associated with the development of acute otitis media (AOM). Childhood infections, such as measles, whooping cough and scarlet fever, may also be implicated. Although many upper respiratory infections are viral in origin, secondary bacterial infection often supervenes, and in acute otitis media, streptococci, staphylococci or pneumococci may be found. The infection involves the mucosal membrane of the whole middle ear cleft, i.e. Eustachian tube, tympanic cavity, attic, aditus, antrum and mastoid air cells. This generalised inflammation results in the formation of pus (Fig. 1.10a, b and c) which exerts pressure on the tympanic membrane causing severe otalgia. Eventually, the tympanic membrane ruptures, with release of pus and relief of pain.

Clinical features

The affected child complains of severe pain in the ear. He will by pyrexial and may appear quite toxic. Examination of the tympanic membrane reveals it to be red and bulging. Adequate analgesia in appropriate doses will alleviate the most distressing symptom of pain.

Treatment and nursing care

Aspirin, if used, will also help to bring down the pyrexia and relieve pain. The local application of warmth by a protected hot water bottle may also be soothing. Great care must be taken in using hot water bottles or heat pads with children. Water hot enough to scald should be avoided and the bottle should be kept covered. Nasal decongestant drops, such as 0.5% ephedrine or xylometazoline HCL 0.1% (Table 2.2), will help to reduce oedema of the Eustachian tubal mucosa and encourage normal middle ear ventilation. It will also enable the patient to breathe through his nose and so prevent drying of the mouth. Penicillin is the antibiotic of choice in the first instance. If the inflammation does not resolve with this antibiotic, an alternative antibiotic with a broader spectrum should be used. Vigorous treatment is required as the complications can

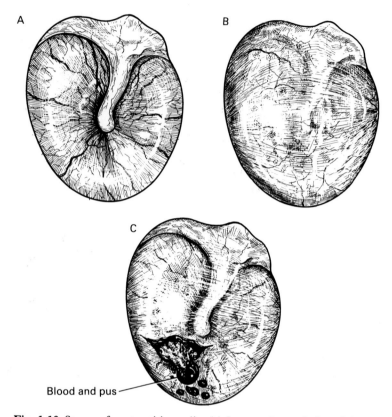

Fig. 1.10 Stages of acute otitis media: (a) Increased vascularity of the tympanic membrane (b) Tense bulging tympanic membrane. Loss of normal anatomical features (c) Large rupture in tympanic membrane in the pars tensa.

be very serious. Whilst pyrexial and toxic the patient requires all the normal care for the febrile patient. Bed rest is advisable until the pyrexia settles. A good fluid intake should be encouraged and particular attention paid to oral hygiene.

If the tympanic membrane ruptures, aural toilet should be performed. This should be repeated as often as is considered necessary. The canal should not be packed, but a small piece of cotton wool can be placed at the external meatus to soak up any discharge and prevent contamination of clothing. This should be changed when aural toilet is performed. A swab for bacterial culture and sensitivity should be taken. Nose and throat swabs may also be taken. The nurse should be careful to prevent water from running into the canal until the perforation has healed completely.

Parents should be reassured that complete resolution of the infection will occur, provided that a complete course of antibiotic therapy is given. The need to take the full course must be emphasised to the parents. Ruptures of the tympanic membrane in these circumstances usually heal spontaneously and this can be checked at follow-up. It may be necessary for a child to have his adenoids removed at a later date, especially if attacks of acute otitis media are recurrent.

Complications of acute middle ear infection

In acute otitis media the mucosa of the mastoid antrum and air cells is infected. If the infection is sufficiently virulent, it progresses to involve the bone of the mastoid air cells. Bone destruction leads to the formation of an abscess cavity in the mastoid which results in swelling behind the pinna which may be pushed forwards. As with abscess formation elsewhere, the treatment is surgical drainage. This is achieved by the operation of cortical mastoidectomy, performed under antibiotic cover (Fig. 1.15).

Facial nerve paralysis may develop in acute otitis media if the bony facial canal is deficient and the nerve is exposed to acute infection. Recovery follows appropriate antibiotic treatment of the acute infection.

Chronic middle ear infection

There are two main types of chronic middle ear infection.

Mucosal type

This type is characterised by the presence of a perforation in the pars tensa of the tympanic membrane. Perforations vary greatly in size and position (Figs. 1.11a and b) and, while they may be dry, they are often associated with a mixed bacterial infection of the middle ear producing intermittent discharge. Recurrent exacerbations are often caused by water entering the ear whilst the patient is washing his hair or swimming or diving into infected water. Apart from discharge the patient may also complain of deafness. This may be due to the perforation itself or may be a result of damage to the ossicular chain. In particular, the incudo-stapedial joint is prone to the effects of chronic infection, with erosion of the long process of the incus producing discontinuity of the ossicular chain (Fig. 1.12).

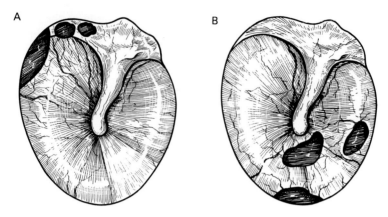

Fig. 1.11 Chronic suppurative otitis media: (a) 'Dangerous perforations (b) 'Safe' perforations.

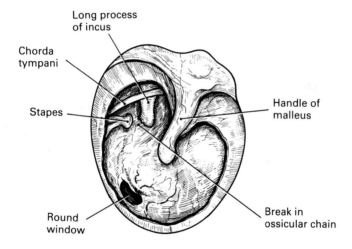

Fig. 1.12 Sub-total perforation showing ossicular discontinuity.

Treatment

The aim of treatment is to seal off the middle ear cavity by using a graft of muscle fascia or dura to close the perforation in the operation of myringoplasty. Reconstruction of the ossicular chain may be carried out at the same time or at a subsequent procedure called an ossiculoplasty (Fig. 1.13). The combination of these operative procedures will prevent further infection and will also restore hearing to normal.

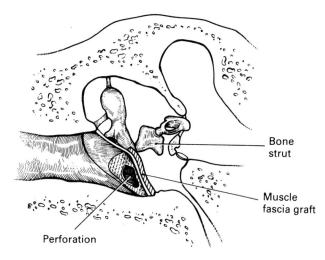

Fig. 1.13 Ossiculoplasty and myringoplasty.

Cholesteatomatous chronic suppurative otitis media

In this type of infection, the perforation of the tympanic membrane occurs posteriorly or superiorly in the pars flaccida (Fig. 1.14). A cholesteatoma, which is an accumulation of epithelial debris, develops; this then becomes infected by a mixture of aerobic and

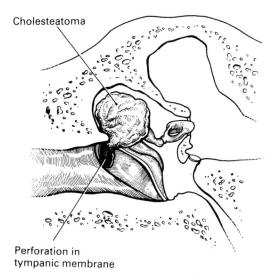

Fig. 1.14 Cholesteatoma formation in the middle ear.

anaerobic bacteria producing a characteristically foul smelling discharge. The cholesteatoma may extend into the attic, antrum and mastoid air cells and remain undetected until the development of serious complications which will be discussed in a later section (p. 26). In common with the mucosal type of infection, cholesteatomatous chronic infection will also cause serious damage to the ossicles.

Treatment

The aims of treatment are to eradicate all infected material from the middle ear and mastoid air cells and to preserve, if possible, good hearing. The operation of mastoidectomy is the most usual procedure. In this operation, bone is removed to expose the attic, antrum and mastoid air cells (Fig. 1.15a and b). Careful eradication of all of the cholesteatoma will ensure that serious complications do not occur. A bony mastoid cavity is left which can be easily inspected at follow-up. Since cholesteatoma is very liable to recur, frequent follow-up is desirable. Unfortunately, control of the disease process may result in reduced levels of hearing, since parts of the ossicular chain may have to be removed to achieve complete clearance of the cholesteatoma. However, once eradication has been achieved, attempts can be made to reconstruct the tympanic membrane and ossicular chain. The term tympanoplasty is used to describe this technique which embraces both myringoplasty and ossiculoplasty.

Complications of chronic suppurative otitis media

Reference to the anatomical relationships of the middle ear cavity and mastoid air cells (Fig. 1.16) illustrates the potential complications which may arise from the spread of chronic suppurative otitis media. Intracranial spread poses the most serious threat to life. Meningitis and intracranial abscess formation in the temporal lobe or cerebellum may occur. This complication requires the combined efforts of otolaryngologist and neurosurgeon to drain the abscess. Intensive antibiotic therapy and full supportive measures are essential. For details of the nursing care a textbook on neurological/neurosurgical nursing should be consulted (see Further reading on p. 204). The lateral venous sinus lies in close relationship with the mastoid air cells and involvement of it produces a life-threatening thrombophlebitis (Fig. 1.16). Fortunately, these complications are rare nowadays, as adequate measures to treat the chronic infection can be taken to prevent them

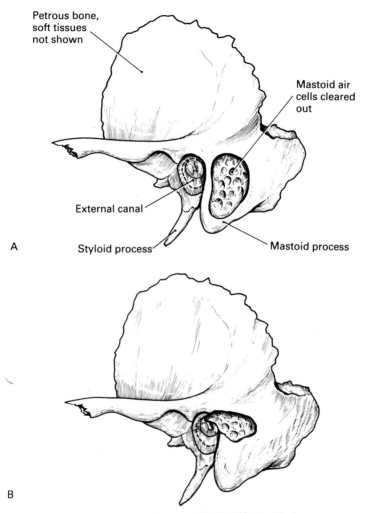

Petrous bone,
soft tissues
not shown

Mastoid air
cells cleared
out

External canal

Mastoid process

A   Styloid process

B

Fig. 1.15 (a) Cortical mastoidectomy (b) Modified radical
mastoidectomy. Healthy parts of middle ear cavity left so that hearing
may be retained.

arising. The facial nerve is also vulnerable if its bony canal is
deficient or if it is eroded. A facial palsy or paralysis is the visible
manifestation of this.

Otosclerosis

In this condition (Fig. 1.17), there is formation of new bone around
the footplate of the stapes, causing this structure to become fixed

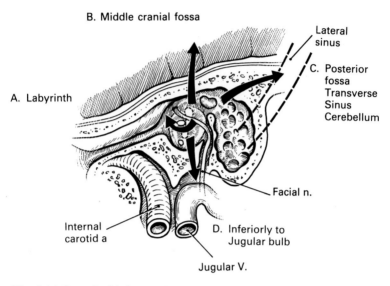

B. Middle cranial fossa

Lateral sinus

C. Posterior fossa Transverse Sinus Cerebellum

A. Labyrinth

Facial n.

Internal carotid a

D. Inferiorly to Jugular bulb

Jugular V.

Fig. 1.16 Spread of infection from middle ear cavity.

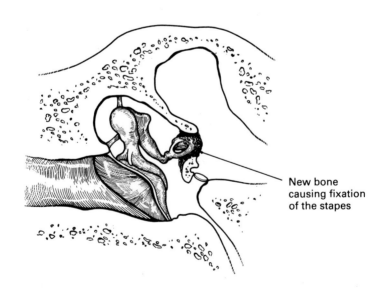

New bone causing fixation of the stapes

Fig. 1.17 Otosclerosis.

and, therefore, unable to transmit sound vibrations to the inner ear. There is a gradual deterioration in hearing which is usually bilateral. It is a common cause of conductive deafness in young adults. The condition is progressive and is often exacerbated by pregnancy. There is usually a strong family history of the disease.

Treatment

Many patients happily accept treatment by means of a hearing aid. Alternatively, some patients are helped more by an operation called a stapedectomy (Fig. 1.18). In this procedure part of the stapes is removed, leaving only the footplate behind. A small hole is drilled in the footplate of the stapes. A teflon prosthesis, shaped like the wire part of a coathanger, is then hooked over the long process of the incus and slotted in to fit neatly in the hole in the footplate. This enables the ossicles to vibrate more freely once more, so allowing sound to be transmitted along the prosthesis to the cochlea. The pre- and post-operative care of patients requiring ear surgery is described below.

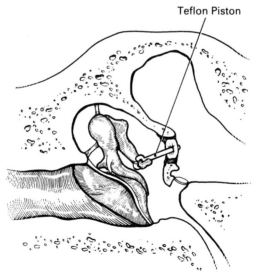

Teflon Piston

Fig. 1.18 Stapedectomy.

Skull fractures

Fractures of the temporal bone may involve the roof of the bony external canal, the roof of the middle ear cavity and extend medially into the petrous part of the temporal bone. Tearing of the skin of the external canal and the tympanic membrane produces bleeding from the ear. This sign following a head injury, may indicate a fracture of this area, even in the absence of positive X-ray evidence.

A compound fracture in this area means that the dura mater has been torn and cerebro-spinal fluid leaks from the ear. This is potentially a very serious complication, since a pathway for infection has been established between the external canal and middle ear to the subarachnoid space. In dealing with this type of injury, nurses must be alert to the possibility of cerebro-spinal otorrhoea and report any slight watery discharge to the doctor. The doctor will prescribe an antibiotic as a prophylaxis against infection (meningitis and/or cerebral abscess), as these are very serious conditions when they arise. The cerebro-spinal fluid leak will generally cease within 7–10 days, so that the problem of infection remains until the dura and overlying tissues heal. Surgical intervention may be necessary. Full neurological observations of conscious level should be carried out half hourly, and the temperature recorded four hourly. Aural toilet should be carried out once or twice daily to keep the external canal clean and so minimise the risk of local infection. Severe damage to the middle ear structures will require to be treated surgically. Unfortunately, damage to the cochlea, acoustic nerve and facial nerve is not usually reversible, so that permanent hearing loss or facial palsy may be a problem. In the case of facial nerve damage, measures may have to be taken to protect the cornea, for example, by using spectacles with a side guard.

Tumours of the ear

The skin of the pinna and the external canal may be the site of squamous cell carcinoma, presenting as an ulcerating bleeding sore which may be painful. Treatment is by a combination of surgery and radiotherapy. Carcinomata of the middle ear and mastoid are thankfully less common since such tumours are difficult to treat and have a poor prognosis.

Diseases of the inner ear

Deafness resulting from disease processes involving the cochlea and acoustic nerves present major difficulties in management since, for the most part, little can be offered in the way of treatment. This form of deafness is called sensorineural and there are many causes. The commoner problems deserve mention.

(a) *Congenital deafness*. This may occur as an inherited condition, or as a result of drugs or infection during pregnancy especially the first twelve weeks, or from trauma or anoxia at birth.

(b) *Infection*. Viral infections such as measles, mumps, influenza or herpes may all result in sensorineural deafness.

(c) *Drugs*. Many different preparations may cause deafness. Two groups of drugs, in particular, are worthy of mention:
(i) the amino glycoside group of antibiotics which includes streptomycin, neomycin, gentamicin and tobramicin. The last two preparations are very ototoxic and administration must be controlled by daily estimations of serum levels in the blood.
(ii) Loop diuretics frusemide and ethnacrynic acid are two which are often prescribed. Frusemide, if administered rapidly in large doses, is very liable to cause sensorineural deafness.

(d) *Effects of age*. Hearing declines slowly throughout adult life. The term applied to this type of deafness, common in old age, is presbyacusis.

(e) *Noise*. Exposure to excessive noise levels for prolonged periods is all too sadly a common, though preventable, cause of deafness. There are now legal requirements in force to try and prevent deafness occurring in occupations in which it was once a serious problem. The law in this area is difficult to enforce, and, as loss of hearing only becomes serious after prolonged exposure, the damage is often done before positive steps to prevent it have been taken. Employers may fail to provide ear defenders, acceptable to the person at risk. Health education, public information films and campaigns to encourage the use of ear protection are a constant need. The world we live in is becoming noisier every day, putting more people at risk. Apart from loss of hearing, noise affects the quality of our lives, causing stress and ill health, even if the cause is not always clearly recognised.

(f) *Trauma*. Fractures of the base of the skull may damage the acoustic nerves or the cochlea, with permanent deafness being the outcome in some cases.

Giddiness

There are many causes of giddiness, and few people at one time or other will not have experienced a transient unsteadiness on sudden movement. In some people, the dysequilibrium is much more persistent and may indeed be so severe as to be a real handicap. When severe giddiness of this nature is experienced it is usually referred to as 'vertigo'.

Other general causes apart from disturbance in the ear arise from the circulatory, central nervous and endocrine systems and other toxic factors.

Many investigations may be required to establish the cause, though in quite a large number of people it may not be possible to identify the reasons.

Treatment

Treatment is aimed at treating any underlying cause, and referral to neurologists and general physicians is quite common. There are drugs which act as labyrinthine sedatives and these can sometimes be of great help in relieving the symptoms. Prochlorperazine and cinnarizine are two such drugs (Table 1.1).

Ménière's disease

This is a disease in which there is a serious disorder of the vestibular and cochlear apparatus.

There are three main symptoms the patient complains of: giddiness and vomiting, deafness and tinnitus. Initially, attacks may be intermittent with long remissions, but later they become more frequent and progressive.

Treatment

Treatment in an acute attack is bed rest. The patient must lie very still and avoid sudden movements of the head. Intramuscular injections of phenobarbitone or chlorpromazine in quite large doses will usually bring about some relief. Because spontaneous remissions occur, it is difficult to provide satisfactory treatment.

The various measures tried indicate our lack of knowledge of the exact cause of the condition. These include salt and fluid restrictions, vasodilator drugs and diuretics. Antihistamine drugs are frequently employed and these may relieve the distressing giddiness and vomiting. Various surgical procedures have been tried, though these are usually reserved for those people in whom medical treatment has failed.

Table 1.1 Preparation acting on the labyrinth

Trade name	Approved name	Presentation	Dose range	Indications
Avomine	Promethazine theoclate	25 mg Tabs	1 tablet 2–3 times per day	Nausea, vomiting, vertigo, motion sickness
Dramamine	Dimenhydrinate	50 mg Tabs	1–2 tablets three times per day	Vertigo, nausea and vomiting
Serc	Betahistine HCL	8 mg Tabs	8–16 mg three times per day	Meniere's syndrome
Stemetil	Prochlorperazine maleate	5 mg Tabs	Up to six tablets per day	Vertigo due to Meniere's disease, other labyrinthine disorders, nausea and vomiting, migraine
Stugeron	Cinnarizine	15 mg Tabs	15–30 mg three times per day	Vestibular disorders, motion sickness
Torecan	Thiethylperazine	6.33 mg Tabs	1 tablet two to three times daily	Nausea, vertigo, vomiting
Valoid	Cyclizine HCL	50 mg Tabs 50 mg/ml INJ	50 mg up to three times daily	Vomiting and nausea, vertigo and labyrinthine disorders
Vertigon Spansule	Prochlorperazine	10 mg and 15 mg sustained release capsules	10–15 mg once or twice daily	Vertigo, nausea, vomiting, minor mental and emotional disturbances

All of the preparations listed must be prescribed by a doctor. The doses listed must be for adults only. Many of the preparation have a sedative effect and may produce a marked drowsiness. This may be a troublesome side-effect in some patients. Patients must be advised about driving or using industrial machinery while receiving these drugs. Other common side-effects include headache, blurred vision, tinnitus, sleep disturbance, gastro-intestinal upset and urinary retention in susceptible patients. Side-effects often subside and become less troublesome after a few days.

Deafness

From the preceding discussion it will be appreciated that there are many causes of deafness. They are classified into main groups; conductive and sensorineural.

Conductive deafness

Diseases affecting the external canal, tympanic membrane and/or the middle ear cavity cause this form of deafness (Tables 1.2 and 1.3). Because these areas are surgically accessible, this type of deafness is treatable by surgery. Often, however, simple amplification by means of a hearing aid may prove a very effective alternative solution.

Table 1.2 Causes of childhood deafness

Congenital	Acquired
Hereditary deafness	Viral infections (measles, mumps, meningitis)
Maternal rubella	Serous otitis media
Drugs in pregnancy e.g. Thalidomide	Acute suppurative otitis media
Hypoxia	Chronic suppurative otitis media
Rhesus incompatibility Idiopathic	

Table 1.3 Causes of adult deafness

Conductive	Sensorineural
External canal wax otitis externa foreign body	Age (presbyacusis) Trauma Noise trauma
Tympanic membrane perforation	Ototoxic drugs
Middle ear ossicular discontinuity (chronic infection/trauma) otosclerosis serous otitis media tumour	Infection (influenza, measles) Syphilis Acoustic neuroma

Sensorineural

As the name suggests, this type of deafness results from damage to the sensory organ (the cochlea) and to the eighth cranial nerve (acoustic nerve) and central neural pathways. In general, surgery has little to offer in the management of such problems. The commonest type of sensorineural deafness is due to age and is given the name presbyacusis.

It is unfortunate that deafness is so prevalent within the community. Much remains to be done to pinpoint and avoid many of the causes and to improve on the early diagnosis and management of established cases. The effects of the affliction differ from one age group to another.

Infants

It is extremely important for everyone involved in the care of infants to appreciate the serious consequences which result from deafness in this age group. Early diagnosis will ensure that measures are taken to allow normal educational, social and emotional development. Even the vaguest suspicion that a child may have impaired hearing justifies thorough investigation and it is, therefore, important to recognise those infants who may be particularly at risk.

Genetic deafness may form part of a well-recognised syndrome. Prenatal factors may be implicated, especially rubella infection during the first 12 weeks of pregnancy and jaundice resulting from Rhesus incompatability. Hypoxia during birth and infections such as meningitis are also aetiological factors. There are, therefore, identifiable groups of children who are 'at risk' and who therefore merit special attention. In other cases, the mother will often notice the problem during the early months of the child's life: her impression will almost certainly be correct.

Normal speech development requires normal hearing. Failure to progress normally with speech is, therefore, a further indication for a full assessment of hearing.

Children

In children of school age the commonest cause of deafness is serous otitis media, usually associated with upper respiratory tract infection (Table 1.2). It is worth emphasising the intermittent nature of this condition, and once it has been diagnosed teachers should be informed so that problems with schooling may be avoided.

It is possible for partial loss of hearing to result from childhood illnesses such as measles or mumps. Unilateral deafness or deafness affecting only particular sound frequencies may remain undetected until routine testing is performed at school.

Adults

The main causes of adult deafness are listed in Table 1.3.

Many of the causes of adult deafness have been mentioned in previous sections. It is certain that the nurse will encounter many patients, both in the community and in hospital, who suffer from varying degrees of deafness. The elderly present special problems, often because they feel embarrassed by their handicaps and do not wish to feel a burden on those who care for them. Difficulty with communication only adds to their distress. Their particular type of deafness often only affects the higher sound frequencies and this reduces their ability to understand consonants. Lower pitched sounds, e.g. vowels, may still be heard well. As a result, simply raising one's voice may have little effect. Face to face conversation with a slightly raised voice and slow, distinct speech in a quiet environment is important. Slow, distinct speech emphasises the consonants and also allows ease of lip reading for the patient. The profoundly deaf can be provided with a notebook and pencil. Communication with any deaf patient is possible with a little understanding and patience.

Many elderly patients will have a hearing aid (see Appendix 1, p. 101). The commonest variety is the ear level aid (Fig. 1.19). This consists of a mould to fit in to the ear., connected by a short length of tubing to a combined microphone and amplifier which sits behind the ear. Its unobtrusive appearance makes it cosmetically acceptable. However, some patients with rheumatoid arthritis, or weakness in their hands, may lack the manual dexterity to insert and adjust the aid (Fig. 1.20a and b). For these people, a body worn aid may be a more suitable alternative.

A simple check by the nurse of the following points will show whether the hearing aid is functioning or not.

(i) The plastic casing of the amplifier should be checked for damage: the tubing should not be kinked and the mould should not be blocked by wax.

(ii) Switching on will produce a loud whistling noise known as 'feedback' if the batteries are working. If this noise is not present then the batteries should be replaced.

(iii) The patient should be able to insert the mould to ensure a neat fit in the ear and adjust the volume control to a suitable level.

Table 1.4 Aural (external ear) preparations

Trade name	Approved name constituents type of presentation	Dose range	Indications/uses
Cerumol	Paradichlorobenzene 2% Chlorbutor 5% Turpentine oil 10%	Instill 5 drops, leave for 10–15 mins before syringing. Alternatively 5 drops for 3 days.	Removal of ear wax.
Chloromycetin	Chloramphenicol (drops) 10%	1–2 drops two to three times daily.	Chronic otorrhoea, suppurative otitis media, infection or fenestration and mastoid operation cavities.
Framygen	Framycetin sulph. (drops) 0.5%	4 drops three to four times daily.	Otitis externa.
Genticin	Gentamicin (as sulphate) (drops) 0.3%	2–4 drops three to four times daily and at night.	Bacterial ear infections.
Neo-cortef	Neomycin sulph. 0.5% Hydrocortisone acetate (drops) 1.5%	1–2 drops two to three times daily.	Otitis externa.
Otosporin	Polymixin B sulph. 10 000 units Neomycin sulph. 0.5% Hydrocortisone (drops) 1%	3 drops initially. 3 drops three to four times daily. Insert soaked wick, keeping it saturated.	Bacterial infections and inflammation of outer ear.
Canestan	Clotrimazole 1% in Polythylene glycol soln.	Apply sparingly 2–3 drops daily.	Fungal infection of the outer ear.

All external (aural) preparations must be prescribed by a doctor. The doses listed above are for adults only. Many and whenever you are unsure of a preparation, its uses and side-effects.

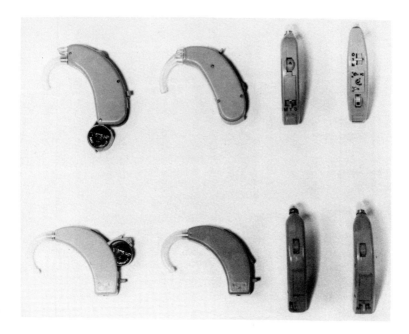

Fig. 1.19 Selection of hearing aids worn behind the ear. Top row: forward facing microphone. Bottom row: lower placed microphone.

The nursing care of patients with ear disorders

Introduction

The majority of people with ear disorders are seen by the general practitioner and prescribed treatment for self-medication. Others are referred to the otolaryngology clinic for further investigation and treatment. Of these, a small number are admitted to hospital for more elaborate investigations and for more intensive medical and surgical treatment.

Pre-operative care

Patients requiring surgery will usually be admitted the day before the operation. On admission, the doctor will examine the patient and assess his/her fitness for surgery. Most ear surgery in the United Kingdom is performed under general anaesthesia. Surgery

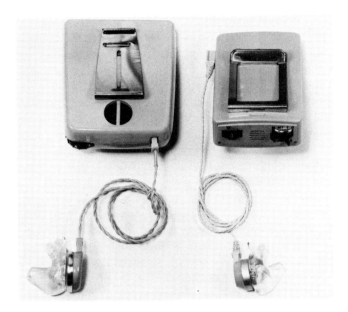

A

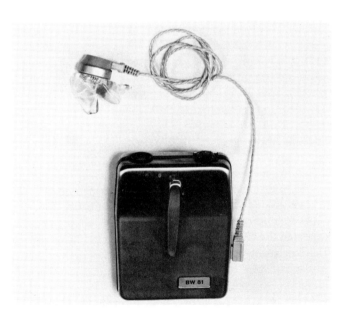

B

Fig. 1.20 (a) Standard National Health Service hearing aids—complete with ear moulds
(b) National Health Service high power hearing aid—designed for people with serious hearing loss.

is only performed under local anaesthesia if general anaesthesia is too risky for the patient. Because of the expertise of anaesthetists, few patients are likely to be at risk from general anaesthesia. It is important that the patient is free from infection and, in particular, that there is no evidence of rhinitis or sinusitis.

Taking a nursing history and assessing the patient's condition is the first essential step in planning the patient's care. Actual and potential problems can be identified and planned for. Problems related to the activities of daily living should be identified early and appropriate actions taken to make the patient's stay in hospital as safe and comfortable as is possible.

If a hearing aid is worn, the type of aid should be noted, whether it is worn in the right or left ear and how effective it is. The nurse should take the opportunity to inspect the hearing aid for faults and, if faulty, arrange for it to be serviced.

Communication is an important aspect of any nursing care, and communicating with the deaf or hard of hearing is even more of a challenge. A slight elevation of the voice is usually sufficient. The nursing history should be taken in a side room or office, since patients do not wish their personal and confidential affairs broadcast to the public. (See the section on communicating with the deaf for other details and hints on how to achieve better communication with sufferers of this hidden handicap.)

Preparation for surgery includes those activities discussed in the Introduction (pp. 1–5). More specific preparations depend on the type of operation. Audiometric tests should always be performed on the day before the operation. The results will be used to compare with post-operative test results. X-rays of the middle ear and mastoid area may be required.

The ear to be operated on should be carefully cleansed by the nurse who must be careful not to let fluid run into the external canal. Hair around the ear may need to be shaved (Fig. 1.21) to allow space for the appropriate incision and to allow for the taking of fascia from the temporalis muscle for the graft. After skin cleansing, the hair must be kept away from the ear by hair fixative or clear cellophane tape. Antibiotics may be instilled on the day before the operation. (See the section on Ear drops (p. 47) for details of this.) In certain circumstances, some surgeons may also prescribe systemic antibiotics prophylactically over the operation period. The use of antibiotics, however, in no way diminishes the need for the very highest standards of pre-, peri- and post-operative care. All the normal pre- and post-operative care for surgery under general anaesthesia is given.

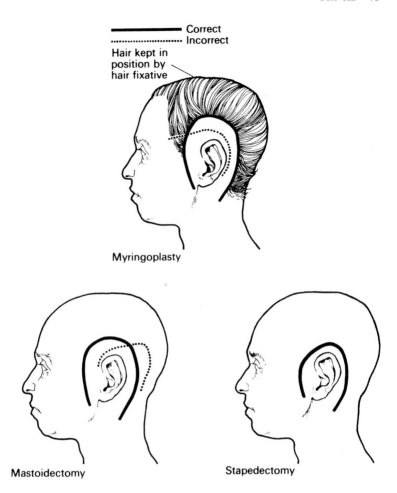

Correct
Incorrect

Hair kept in
position by
hair fixative

Myringoplasty

Mastoidectomy   Stapedectomy

Fig. 1.21 Skin preparations

Post-operative care following ear surgery

Recovery time from anaesthesia will usually be quite short.
However, attention to the patient's airway and vital signs is very
necessary. Positioning is also very important. The patient is nursed
flat, usually with no pillows, having been placed on his side opposite to the ear operated on. The head should be kept still and moved
gently when it has to be. Sudden movements or raising the head
too quickly may cause the patient to experience dizziness and
nausea. All nursing care should be carried out as unhurriedly and
with as little disturbance as possible. As soon as practicable, the

patient should have his hands and face washed and be given a refreshing mouthwash before being changed into his own night-clothes. False teeth, if worn, should be rinsed and replaced at this time. The introduction of one or two pillows will make the patient feel more comfortable. Observations of pulse and blood pressure should continue half-hourly. Following certain types of surgery, such as labyrinthine operations, half-hourly neurological obser-vations may also be required.

Facial nerve damage, either at the time of operation or from oedema or haemorrhage post-operatively, should be checked for by asking the patient to smile or show his teeth. Any facial weakness will then become apparent. If facial palsy is apparent, the surgeon should be informed so that appropriate measures can be made. It may even be necessary for the patient to return to the theatre to have the dressing reviewed. If he is not already on antibiotics, the doctor will most likely prescribe one at this time.

Coughing, sneezing or blowing the nose is not advisable, as pressure transmitted along the Eustachian tube to the middle ear cavity may produce undesirable effects on any reconstructive surgery.

Pain

Local pain around the ear and side of the face may be experienced post-operatively. Analgesics for pain and sedation will initially be prescribed by the anaesthetist. Following this, a simply analgesic such as aspirin or paracetamol will usually be sufficient. Some patients experience a tingling sensation in the tongue if the chorda tympani nerve has been stretched. This latter problem will quickly settle and the patient can be reassured of this.

Giddiness

Following ear surgery some patients may experience dizziness and nausea. The worst of the dizziness can be overcome by gradually raising the patient's head on pillows, and by 24 hours most patients are able to sit up comfortably. Rapid head movements should be discouraged and by 48 hours be patient will be up and about out of bed. The surgeon should be informed if any patient is experi-encing persistent or severe dizziness and/or nausea. Labyrinthine sedatives such as prochlorperazine or cinnarizine may be prescribed (Table 1.1). Experience of dizziness is very variable and each patient needs to be treated as an individual.

Wound care

The nature of dressings, drains and sutures will depend very much on the operation performed (Fig. 1.22a, b and c). Following some of the more extensive mastoid operations, the cavity may be packed for up to seven days. Removal of the packing which has been left in for this period, may require a short general anaesthetic. However, surgeons vary greatly in their approach. Patients who have mastoid cavity packs should have their temperature, pulse and respirations recorded four hourly. The area around the ear should be inspected daily for any signs of inflammation and any complaints of pain or discomfort.

Discharge

Most patients, following ear surgery, will be able to go home in two to three days. Instructions to the patient should begin early. The patient should be instructed on what to do should any problem arise; for example, pain in the ear, dizziness, facial weakness or aural discharge. Some patients may well have to continue using a hearing aid and these must be provided. The patient should be informed about follow-up arrangements. Children who have grommets fitted in their tympanic membrane should avoid swimming, and cotton wool smeared with petrolleum jelly and inserted into the external canal will provide waterproof protection during hair washing and bathing.

Any drugs prescribed should be obtained from the pharmacy prior to the patient's discharge. This will enable the patient to continue his medication until he gets further supplies from his own doctor.

The patient's relatives, where necessary, should be informed of any special care required and of how they can assist in the patient's recovery.

Ear syringing

Syringing the ear is a common nursing procedure. There are three main indications for syringing the external auditory canal, namely, removal of wax, removal of foreign bodies and, more rarely, removal of pus and debris in chronic ear infection.

The most common reason for syringing an ear is to remove wax. Wax or cerumen is produced by specialised apocrine glands to be found in the outer third of the external auditory canal. Its function

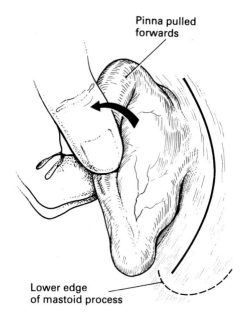

Pinna pulled
forwards

Lower edge
of mastoid process

A

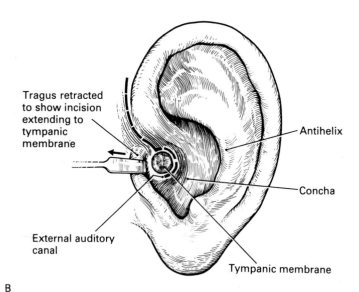

Tragus retracted
to show incision
extending to
tympanic
membrane

Antihelix

Concha

External auditory
canal

Tympanic membrane

B

Fig. 1.22 (a & b) Post-auricular mastoid incision (c) Stapedectomy incision.

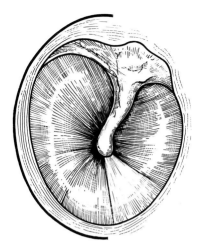

c

is to remove dust and other foreign materials from the canal. In some people, an excessive amount of wax is produced, and this accumulates and eventually blocks the canal causing a conductive deafness. Wax in normal amounts is extruded from the canal by normal chewing movements which 'massage' the cartilaginous outer part of the canal. Sometimes the wax causes a local irritation, inducing the individual to poke his ears and so pushing wax back into the body part of the canal. In addition, if water is allowed to run into the ear when washing it causes the wax to swell. On some occasions, it becomes very hard and impacted. Removal of wax, then, is by no means a simple procedure.

Because the wax is often hard and impacted it has to be softened before removal is attempted. The wax can be softened by simple lubricants, such as warm olive or almond oil drops instilled twice a day for 3–4 days. These agents are safe and non-irritant. There are several proprietary cerumenolytic agents available (Table 1.4). These have to be instilled about thirty minutes before syringing. They are very effective at softening and slackening the wax. They should not be used if there is any suspicion that the patient may have a perforated tympanic membrane.

The nurse must never syringe a patient's ear without a doctor prescribing the procedure. There are risks, and contra-indications include dry perforations of the tympanic membrane and acute otitis externa or media.

Various lotions can be used, but plain tap water is perfectly adequate. Some doctors prescribe a 1% sodium bicarbonate solution or normal saline. The lotion must be at body temperature when it is injected into the canal, or convection currents may be set up in the labyrinth if it is too hot or too cold. It is important to use a proper aural syringe as this provides for good control so that risk of damage to the external canal or tympanic membrane is minimised.

The procedure is explained to the patient and reasons are given as to why it is necessary. The patient is best seated in an upright position with his clothes protected by a waterproof cape. The patient can assist by holding the receiver for the return fluid. The temperature should be checked and the syringe filled. The pinna of the ear is pulled upwards and backwards and the nozzle of the syringe is directed towards the roof of the canal (Fig. 1.23). Once the wax of foreign material has been cleared from the canal, it should be inspected to see that it is clean and that no injuries have occurred. The canal can be mopped dry using a Jobson-Horne probe tipped with fluffed cotton wool. If a perforation is discovered on inspection, the doctor will usually prescribe some antibiotic/steroid drops (Table 1.4). Follow-up is essential. Patients who have had

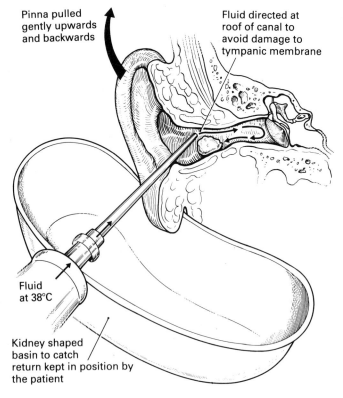

Pinna pulled gently upwards and backwards

Fluid directed at roof of canal to avoid damage to tympanic membrane

Fluid at 38°C

Kidney shaped basin to catch return kept in position by the patient

Fig. 1.23 Syringing the external auditory meatus.

wax impacting the canal for some time will more than likely notice a big improvement in their hearing and be appreciative of the minor inconvenience of the syringing. Patients should be given advice on the care of their ears, especially with regard to the excessive use of cotton buds and too enthusiastic cleaning. The external canal in its structure and production of wax is very well designed to keep itself in good health.

Instillation of ear drops

Ear drops are usually instilled to treat infections. Various topical antibiotics are in common use. Many preparations also have steroids added. Other drops in use are agents which soften wax (Table 1.4).

The drops should be warmed to body temperature before being instilled, as drops that are too hot or cold may set up convection currents in the labyrinth and semi-circular canals which will make the person feel dizzy.

The patient is informed of what is to happen and should be asked to lie on his bed in the lateral position with the ear to be treated uppermost. Only drops specifically prescribed for the patient should be used. The pinna is pulled gently upwards and backwards and the drops instilled as prescribed. Gentle massage of the tragus will ensure the medication flows into the canal. If the patient has a perforation of the tympanic membrane the surgeon may request that the tragus be massaged to ensure that the medication passes all the way along the canal and into the middle ear cavity via the perforation. Where the drops are for infection in which there is discharge, the external canal should be mopped clear of debris before fresh drops are instilled. The patient is best seated upright for this, and after appropriate explanation the pinna is pulled upwards and backwards to straighten the canal so that it can be inspected. A good light is essential. A lamp and head mirror are perhaps best, but they require a good deal of practice for effective use. An auriscope with an appropriate-sized speculum is relatively easy to use. Patients are often expected to instill their own drops on discharge and simple instructions regarding instillation and aural toilet should be given. Failure to do so will often mean that the medication is not used in a satisfactory manner and so is not as effective as it might be.

N.B. To avoid the risk of cross infection, patients with bilateral ear infections should always use a separate bottle of drops for each ear.

Two
The nose

NASAL CAVITY

Applied anatomy and physiology

The nasal cavity is the first part of the respiratory tract. It is enclosed in its upper third by a pair of nasal bones, whilst support in the lower two thirds is provided by two pairs of nasal cartilages: the upper and lower lateral cartilages (Fig. 2.1). The cavity is divided into two airways of equal size by the nasal septum which consists of cartilage anteriorly and bone posteriorly (Fig. 2.2a and b). Deviation of this septum from the midline is a common cause of nasal obstruction.

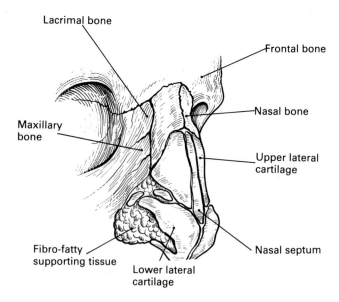

Fig. 2.1 Bony and cartilaginous framework of the nose.

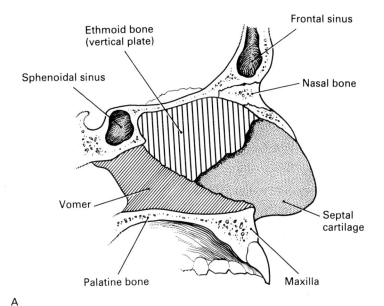

A

B

Fig. 2.2(A) Sagittal sections showing bony and cartilaginous arrangement of the nasal septum. (**B**) Coronal section through nose to show normal position of the nasal septum.

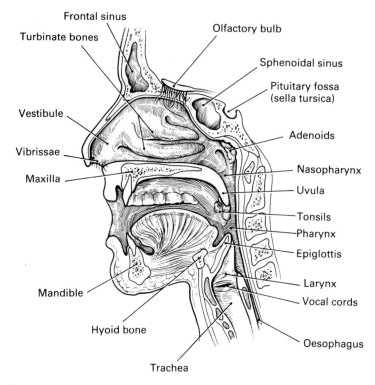

Fig. 2.3 Sagittal section showing lateral walls of nose and pharynx.

The opening of each nostril leads into the vestibule, an area lined by squamous epithelium and containing coarse hairs. The medial wall of each side of the nose is flat and formed by the septum, while the lateral wall is characterised by the projection of three turbinate bones (inferior, middle and superior) (Fig. 2.3). Most of the sinuses drain into the area below the middle turbinate bone. The lacrimal duct carrying excess tears from the eye drain just below the inferior turbinate (Fig. 7.10).

The nasal passages are lined by a mucous membrane of ciliated columnar epithelium which contains many secretory glands and is extremely vascular.

The blood supply to the nose

The anterior and posterior ethmoidal arteries supply the mucous membrane high up in the nose. The naso-palatine artery, a branch of the maxillary artery, supplies the lower part of the back of the

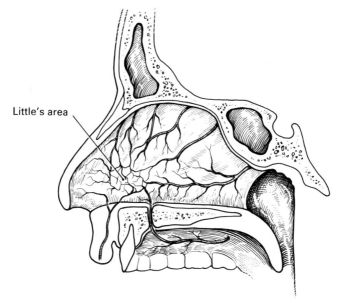

Fig. 2.4 Blood supply to the nasal septum.

nasal cavity. These vessels anastomose at Little's area on each side
of the nasal septum (Fig. 2.4). This is a frequent site for bleeding.

Functions of the nose

The nose functions as the air conditioning unit for the upper and
lower respiratory tract, ensuring that inspired air passes to the lungs
in the correct state. Coarse airborne particles, such as dust, are
trapped in the hairs of the vestibule. Smaller particles, such as
infective agents, adhere to the sticky mucus covering of the nasal
mucosa and are swept back to the nasopharynx by the ciliary
system.

The vascular nasal mucosa, especially over the inferior turbinates, is under the control of the autonomic nervous system and
ensures that cold inspired air is rapidly warmed. At the same time,
the nasal secretions provide humidification and thereby prevent the
air from having a drying effect in the bronchial tree.

Sense of smell

The sense of smell is provided by the terminal fibres of the olfactory
nerve which projects through the cribriform plate (Fig. 2.3).

Bacteriology

A wide variety of bacteria may inhabit the nose. Twenty per cent of normal individuals are carriers of *Staphylococcus aureus* which may be responsible for serious hospital infection. Because of this colonisation, foreign bodies lodged in the nose rapidly become infected and cause nasal discharge. Likewise, nasal packing rapidly becomes infected if measures are not taken to avoid this.

Disorders of the nose

Congenital choanal atresia

Congenital atresia of the posterior part of the nose is caused by the persistence of the bucco-nasal membrane. If the atresia is bilateral, the new born baby soon develops respiratory difficulty and is unable to feed. The persisting membrane must, therefore, be broken down and removed as soon as possible.

Nasal trauma

A blow to the nose may result in cosmetic deformity due to fractures of the nasal bones or deformity of the nasal cartilages. The septum is particularly prone to buckling from trauma, thereby producing nasal obstruction (Fig. 2.5). As a first aid measure, ice applied to the nose may reduce oedema and lessen the tendency for epistaxis. The cosmetic deformity and septal deviation may be

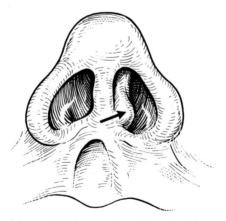

Fig. 2.5 The anterior end of the septal cartilage is dislocated and partially obstructing the nasal vestibule.

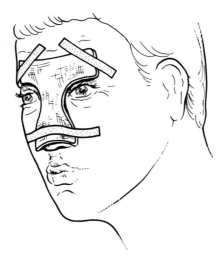

Fig. 2.6 Plaster of Paris splint to support nasal bones after reduction of a fracture.

corrected by manipulation under a general anaesthetic. This is usually done 3–4 days after the injury to give time for any swelling to settle, so allowing accurate assessment of the deformity.

A plaster of Paris (P.O.P.) splint may be applied (Fig. 2.6) to immobilise the reduced fracture. The nursing care following fractures of the nose is similar to that following nasal surgery and details are given below, following a description of the common nasal operations.

Septal deviation

In this condition the nasal septum is deviated from the midline (Fig. 2.7a, b and c). It may be a congenital or developmental abnormality. It is commonly caused, also, by trauma to the nose, in which the nasal bones have been fractured and displaced and not reset properly.

The most usual complaints are those of nasal obstruction, difficulty in breathing through the nose.

Treatment

There are two types of operation commonly performed for this condition; submucous resection (S.M.R.) and septoplasty (Fig. 2.8a and b). The two forms of treatment are often confused by nurses

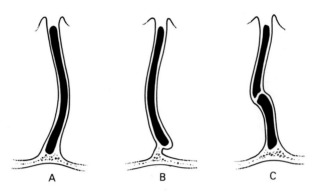

Fig. 2.7 Main causes of deviated nasal septum: (a) Congenital
(b) Dislocation (c) Fracture.

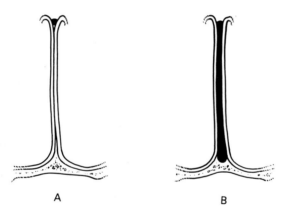

Fig. 2.8 Operations to correct septal deviation: (a) Sub-mucous resection
in which the rigid cartilage has been removed allowing the soft tissues to
come together; (b) Septoplasty—in this procedure the septal cartilage
and bone is remodelled so that it once more lies in the mid-line.

and others. Both procedures involve an approach to the cartilaginous and bony parts of the septum by stripping off the mucosa.
Both involve the removal of parts of the septum. In S.M.R., the
emphasis is on the removal and resection of parts of the septum
causing the deviation (Fig. 2.8a and b). This procedure has been
favoured for many years, but it is criticised because it may result
in removal of parts of the normal support of the nose. In septoplasty, the septum is completely freed and the removal of areas
around its margin may allow it to be repositioned in the midline
(Fig. 2.8a and b). The nursing care following both procedures is

similar and is described below in the section on pre- and post-operative care (p. 68).

Foreign bodies in the nose

Many children insert small foreign bodies into the nose. Delay in recognising the problem results in the child being presented with a unilateral nasal discharge. The object may have been in the nasal cavity for sometime, the child having long since forgotten he had ever pushed it into his nose. The discharge is usually purulent and may be foul smelling. The characteristic feature is that the discharge is from the one nostril only. Removal may be difficult, and to enable a thorough exploration the foreign body is usually removed under a general anaesthetic. The discharge will clear up in a few days and the patient should have no further problems.

Epistaxis

Bleeding from the nose is a very common condition. Whilst for most people it is an annoying incovenience lasting only a few minutes, in others it may be life threatening.

Aetiology

(a) *Bleeding from Little's area* is very common. It is often associated with trauma to the nasal mucosa or upper respiratory infection. It is a common occurrence in children, often the result of 'picking the nose'. Control can be achieved by applying gentle pressure to the cartilaginous part of the nose between the index finger and the thumb (Fig. 2.9). The bleeding is easily controlled, although recurrent episodes may require the offending area to be cauterised using trichloroacetic acid (T.C.A.), silver nitrate or chromic acid. Following cautery, there is often some crusting which children, in particular, may have a tendency to pick off. A local application of petroleum jelly twice a day for a few weeks will help to prevent crusts from forming and allow the epithelium to thicken and heal and so lessen the risk of further episodes. Repeated episodes of epistaxis, even if blood loss is minimal, may lead to anaemia.

(b) *Hypertension.* Epistaxis in middle-aged and elderly people is often due to elevations of the blood pressure. In these circumstances, the bleeding is often from a site at the back of the nose which is difficult to visualise except by direct means.

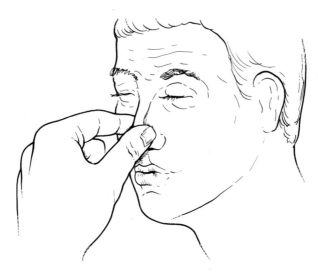

Fig. 2.9 First aid treatment of epistaxis—pressure on the soft cartilaginous part of the nose.

(c) *Haematological disorder.* Abnormal bleeding may be associated with leukaemia, thrombocytopenia and haemophilia. Coagulation defects may arise in chronic liver disease and poorly controlled anticoagulant therapy.

(d) *Hereditary.* A rare disorder of blood vessels, hereditary telangiectasia, usually shows first as epistaxis. The bleeding is usually easily stopped by simple first aid measures. However, if the disorder is not recognised, these patients may be subjected to repeated cauterisation which eventually seriously damages the nasal septum.

(e) *New growths.* Nasal and paranasal tumours may occasionally be the cause of nose bleed. Tumours of this type are not common.

Treatment

If simple first aid measures fail to stop the nose bleeding, the patient should be referred to hospital and may require admission.

In hospital, the initial management is anterior nasal packing, using ribbon gauze impregnated with petrolleum jelly or bismuth iodoform paraffin paste (B.I.P.P.) (Fig. 2.10). Local anaesthetic is provided by lignocaine and adrenaline to allow comfortable pack

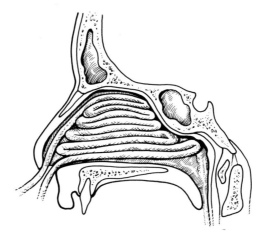

Fig. 2.10 Nasal cavity packed with ribbon gauze.

insertion. This form of packing is left in for 24 hours and will be effective in controlling the bleeding in the majority of patients. Occasionally, however, anterior packing fails to provide control of the bleeding and the technique must be modified to allow for firmer packing.

(a) *Foley catheter insertion.* In this technique, use is made of the balloon of the catheter to provide a firmer base against which to pack the nose. The catheter is inserted along the floor of the nose and when the balloon is sited at the posterior choana it is inflated. The balloon in this position, therefore, allows very firm anterior packing to be achieved. If catheters are inserted in both sides then they may be tied together over the columella. It is important to protect the columella with packing under the catheters to prevent pressure necrosis of the skin (Fig. 2.11).

(b) *Post-nasal pack* (Fig. 2.12a & b). Under a general anaesthetic a gauze pack is inserted into the post-nasal space to allow firm anterior packing. These packs are left in for up to twenty four hours or longer. Frequent observations are required with particular attention being paid to oral hygiene. Antibiotics are usually given, as packing in the nose predisposes the patient to infection.

   In some patients, the bleeding cannot be controlled by any of the methods described, and in these circumstances the vessels supplying the nose have to be ligated, i.e. the anterior ethmoidal and/or maxillary arteries.

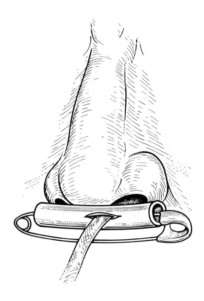

Fig. 2.11 One method of securing nasal pack.

Blood loss from epistaxis may be considerable. Hypovolaemic shock is a real possibility. The patient is confined to bed and is given a sedative to relieve his anxiety. Blood loss is assessed and a blood transfusion given. Intravenous fluids may also be necessary. Half-hourly observations of the pulse and blood pressure are obligatory. In hypertensive patients, anti-hypertensive drugs may be prescribed. The patient and his relatives need reassurance and support as prolonged epistaxis causes considerable anxiety. An iron preparation may be required for a few months to correct any anaemia.

Important points

(a) Reassurance is essential as epistaxis can be a frightening experience.
(b) Cold compresses applied locally in the form of ice packs may help to control bleeding.
(c) The patient should be encouraged to lean forward and discouraged from swallowing any blood as this may cause vomiting.
(d) An attempt should be made to estimate the amount of blood lost.

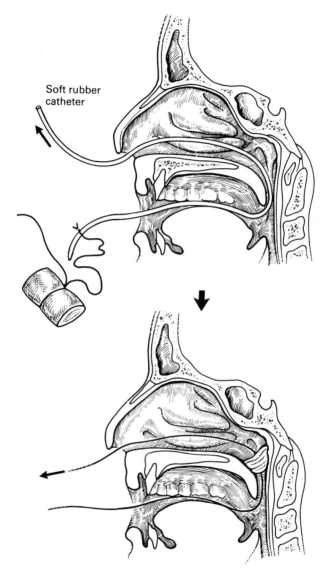

Soft rubber catheter

Fig. 2.12 Insertion of a post-nasal pack.

Allergic rhinitis

Diseases of allergic origin are common in the community, and eczema and asthma form a triad of conditions with allergic rhinitis, all sharing a similar pathogenesis.

Table 2.1 Common allergens

House dust
House dust mite
Grass pollen
Cat fur
Dog hair
Feathers
Moulds
Occupational allergens

While grass pollen and house dust mite are the most likely allergies, there are many others (Table 2.1). Exposure in a sensitive patient causes violent sneezing, watery nasal discharge, irritation to the eyes and nasal obstruction.

The diagnosis is based on a carefully taken medical history and examination. Skin testing will confirm this and may indicate other allergies to which the patient responds.

Simple avoidance of the allergen is the best form of management, but may not always be practicable. Symptomatic relief can be achieved by use of antihistamines or local nasal sprays of steroid, or sodium cromoglycate can be used to prevent attacks.

A course of desensitisation injections is often the only hope of actual cure of the condition, but the results of this form of treatment are not uniformly successful.

Nasal polyps

Nasal polypi (Fig. 2.13) are the end product of prolonged oedema of the nasal mucosa as a result of nasal allergy or chronic sinus infection. They appear in the nose looking rather like bunches of grapes. They are usually multiple, bilateral and look greyish in colour. They have a scanty blood supply, and a characteristic finding is a large quantity of eosinophils, plasma cells and lymphocytes, all suggestive of an allergic type of disorder.

The most common complaint is nasal obstruction, and nasal discharge ranging from mucoid to purulent is frequent. Headaches may also be a feature, especially if there is sinus involvement.

The treatment is surgical removal in the majority of cases. The pre- and post-operation care is similar to that for patients requiring nasal surgery for other reasons, as described below (p. 68). Treatment of the underlying cause, for example chronic sinus infection,

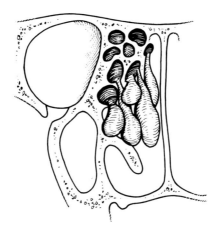

Fig. 2.13 Ethmoidal polyps causing nasal obstruction.

is dealt with in the normal way, as is allergic rhinitis if this is thought to be a predisposing feature.

Regular follow-up should be encouraged as the polyps are liable to recur and are more easily dealt with and less incovenient to the patient if they are treated early.

THE PARANASAL SINUSES

Applied anatomy and physiology

Examination of a human skull will show that there are a number of air spaces surrounding the nose. These are called the paranasal sinuses (Fig. 2.14). The frontal, maxillary and ethmoidal sinuses are paired structures, while the single sphenoid lies under the pituitary fossa (Fig. 2.3). All the sinuses open into the lateral wall of the nose through their ostia, which allow entry of air to ventilate them and drainage of secretions. The sinuses lighten the weight of the skull and give resonance to the voice.

The sinuses have several important anatomical relationships which are of significance to the spread of infection. The floor of the maxillary sinus is closely related to the roots of the upper molar teeth, while its roof separates it from the orbit. The ethmoid sinuses are also in close proximity to the orbit which lies lateral to them. The frontal sinuses lie close to both the orbits and brain.

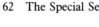

Fig. 2.14 Ostia draining the frontal ethmoidal and antral sinus.

Disorders of the sinuses

Acute sinusitis

Acute sinus infection is usually secondary to viral nasal infections such as coryza (the common cold) or influenza. Secondary bacterial infection by streptococci, pneumococci or staphylococci quickly intervene. The natural resistance of the mucosa is reduced in viral infection and bacteria are quick to exploit this. The maxillary sinus is occasionally involved, by infection spreading from the apices of the molar teeth. The ciliated columnar epithelium of the sinus mucosa responds to the infection by increased mucus production. Swelling of the mucosa quickly closes off the ostia and, as a result, the infected mucus is unable to escape. Progression of the infection can sometimes be particularly virulent and may lead to serious complications.

Complications

(a) Direct spread of the infection from the frontal or ethmoidal sinuses may involve the orbit. Abscess formation in the periorbital tissues puts the eye at risk and, in addition, may spread further to produce intracranial complications.

(b) Intra-cranial infection, including meningitis, intracerebral abscess or superior sagittal sinus thrombophlebitis, may occur.

(c) *Osteomyelitis*—infection may spread to bone. This occurs occasionally in young children as a result of maxillary sinusitis, whilst in adults it is more often secondary to frontal sinusitis.

Clinical features

The symptoms of acute sinus infection usually follow on from upper respiratory tract infection or dental disease. Pain occurs, the site of which depends on the sinus involved. Maxillary sinus infection causes facial pain, frontal sinusitis causes supraorbtial pain and ethmoidal involvement causes pain between the eyes. Nasal obstruction is a common feature of sinusitis, regardless of which sinuses are involved. Discharge may be present, although it is not excessive if the ostia draining the sinuses are blocked.

The patient looks and feels unwell, is pyrexial and usually complains of general malaise. Local tenderness may be elicited and mucopurulent material may be seen in the nose.

Treatment

Treatment consists of nasal decongestant drops (Table 2.2) which reduce the mucosal oedema, allowing the ostia to open and permit drainage. An antibiotic such as penicillin will usually be appropriate. Swabs can be sent for culture and sensitivity if the infection does not respond to the penicillin. Pain relief is essential and can usually be achieved by aspirin or paracetamol. If the condition does not resolve, an antral lavage (see p. 65) may be required. Abscess formation demands immediate surgical intervention under appropriate broad spectrum antibiotic cover. Swabs should be sent for culture and sensitivity. Failure to treat a sinus abscess properly may result in spread of the infection to the orbit or to the brain.

Nursing care

The patient requires all the care normally given to a febrile patient. He should be confined to bed in a warm well-ventilated room. A liberal fluid intake of at least three litres per day for an adult should be given. Particular attention is given to oral hygiene. Local meas-

Table 2.2 Nasal preparations

Trade name	Approved name constituents type of preparation	Dose range	Indications/uses
Afrazine	Oxymetazoline HCL 0.15 mg (spray or drops)	2–3 drops or sprays in each nostril twice daily	Nasal congestion
Dexa-rhinaspray	Tramazoline HCL 0.12 mg Dexamethasone 21 130 nicotinate 0.02 mg Neomycin sulph. 0.1 mg (per metered dose aerosol)	1 application in each nostril up to maximum 6 times in 24 hours	Allergic rhinitis
Otrivine	Xylometazoline HCL 0.1% (drops or sprays)	2–3 drops or 1–2 sprays in each nostril 2–3 times daily	Nasal congestion
Rynacrom M	Sodium cromoglycate 20% Solution with metered dose pump (also drops or spray and insufflation capsules)	Adults and children 1 dose to each nostril 6 times daily	Allergic rhinitis, hay fever

All nasal preparations must be prescribed by a doctor. The doses listed are for adults only. Many preparations are not recommended for paediatric use. Many of the products listed contain sympathomimetic amines and must not be used over prolonged periods or indiscriminantly; such usage may lead to rebound symptoms on withdrawal. Topical applications of antihistamines may produce skin sensitization and subsequent eczematous and other eruptions. Nurses should encourage patients to comply strictly with the treatment as prescribed.

ures such as steam inhalations are soothing and give additional symptomatic relief. In a day or two the patient will have recovered sufficiently to be up and about. He should remain indoors and avoid extremes of temperature and, of course, complete his antibiotic and any other therapy as prescribed.

Chronic sinus infection

Several factors may be implicated in chronic low grade sinus infection. These include: (a) inadequate treatment of acute infection, (b) poor ventilation and drainage of the sinus because of septal deviation or polyps, (c) pollution by cigarette smoke and other industrial pollutants, (d) allergic nasal disease. Any one or a combination of these may result in chronic sinusitis. It is usual to find a mixture of pathogenic bacteria in this type of longstanding infection. The sinus mucosa becomes hypertrophied and sometimes polypoidal (see above) (Fig. 2.13).

Clinical features

The main clinical features are nasal discharge, post-nasal discharge (post-nasal drips) and huskiness of the voice. The condition is often long standing, one of the main aggravating factors being excessive smoking.

The treatment is a course of broad spectrum antibiotics such as tetracycline combined with nasal decongestants (Table 2.2). This may effect a cure. The patient, if a smoker, should be encouraged to stop and should, if possible, avoid dry smoky or dusty atmospheres. In many patients the disorder is extremely refractory and other more drastic measures are therefore required. The most commonly involved sinuses are the maxillary sinuses. The ostia in these are badly located (Fig. 2.14); as a result, they do not drain adequately. Because of this, it sometimes helps to wash out the sinuses, a procedure called an antral lavage.

Antral lavage

This procedure is done for both treatment and diagnosis. It involves the introduction of a trocar and cannula (Fig. 2.15) into the maxillary (or antral) sinus to obtain a specimen (proof puncture) or to wash out infected material from the sinus (antral lavage) (Fig. 2.16). The principles of the procedure are shown in the diagram which demonstrates how the natural ostia of the sinus are made use of.

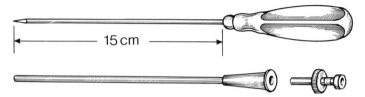

Fig. 2.15 Lichwitz trocar and cannula.

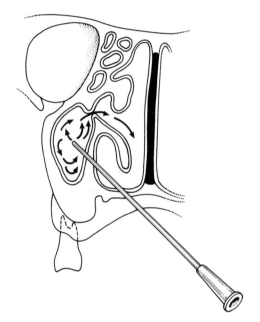

Fig. 2.16 Position of Lichwitz trocar in the antral lavage.

The procedure should be carefully explained to the patient without alarming him. The nostrils should be cleansed before the procedure. To remove crusting and dried-on secretions, a weak sodium bicarbonate or hydrogen peroxide solution can be used. The patient should be seated comfortably and a good light is essential. Using dressed orange sticks dipped in the chosen solution, the nostrils are gently cleaned to remove all dried-on secretions. Care must be taken not to damage the nasal mucosa. Infection of the vestibule is common and the cleaning action may cause some discomfort or pain. Either a topical anaesthetic or a local anaesthetic can be used. The patient should be sitting upright with his head supported by a nurse. This is necessary as considerable force may be necessary to introduce the cannula. It also lessens the risk of complications. Once the trocar and cannula are in position, the trocar is removed and a Higginson's syringe is attached to the cannula. The sinus can then be irrigated using sterile normal saline. The fluid is pumped into the sinus by gently squeezing the bulb of the Higginson's syringe. The fluid returns via the pattern's nose and a suitable receptacle should be provided to catch this. The clothes should be protected by a waterproof cape. The nurse should observe the patient carefully as he may feel pain, especially when the cannula is introduced.

On completion of the irrigation the patient rests quietly for a few hours. Observations should be made for bleeding or haematoma formation. When the effects of the local anaesthetic have worn off, any pain can be treated with a simple analgesic. All other treatment being given concurrently, such as inhalations, decongestants and antibiotics, should be given as prescribed. If the procedure is done in the Day Bed Area or Out-Patients Department, adequate instructions should be given to the patient regarding continuing treatment and other practical measures he can take to help resolve the condition. Poor compliance with therapy, especially antibiotic, may be a factor in the condition's refractory nature. Over-use of decongestant drops is, of course, undersirable as this may lead on to atrophic rhinitis.

Intranasal antrostomy

In this procedure, a wide opening is made under the inferior turbinate bone into the antro-nasal wall. The purpose of this opening is for washing out the sinus. The procedure is carried out under a general anaesthetic.

Radical antrostomy (Caldwell-Luc)

This is a more extensive procedure in which the maxillary sinus is opened through the canine fossa (Fig. 2.17). This allows the sinus to be viewed directly so that the condition of the mucosa can be assessed. If need be, the mucous membrane may be removed in part or in whole. The procedure is done under a general anaesthetic. This has the advantage that the pharynx and respiratory passage can be isolated using a pack in the pharynx and an endo-tracheal tube. This prevents any infected material reaching the lungs. No packing

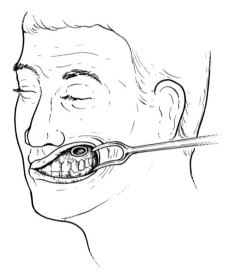

Fig. 2.17 Caldwell-Luc antrostomy.

is used, though if bleeding is persistent a small gauze pack soaked in paraffin can be left in for several hours. The wound in the mouth is closed with a catgut suture. Some blood-stained serum should be expected for a day or two. On the second post-operation day, the sinus is washed out using normal saline or boric lotion. This may be repeated daily for a few days. Steam inhalations are given three times daily to reduce nasal congestion. An oily spray or drops of liquid paraffin are administered to prevent crusting on the nasal mucosa.

Nasal surgery

Pre-operative care

The patient requiring nasal surgery will usually be admitted the day before the operation. The only special pre-operative investigation will probably be X-rays of the nasal bones and sinuses. Patients should receive all the usual care of someone having surgery under general anaesthesia.

If packs are to be inserted during the operation, the patient should be told about these. It must be explained to him that he will not be able to breathe through his nose and that he will have to breathe through his mouth. In the case of operations for deviated nasal septum he should be warned that because of swelling the full

benefits of the operation may not be immediately apparent and that
it may be several weeks before improvement is really noticeable.
Most nasal surgery is performed under a general anaesthetic.
However, because of the vascularity of the nasal mucosa, pre-
operative measures to reduce intranasal bleeding are of value. The
method described by Moffat is in common use. In this method a
mixture of lignocaine and adrenaline is prepared and introduced
into the nose. The lignocaine anaesthetises the mucous membrane
and the adrenaline constricts the blood vessels. Moving the patient
into different positions allows the local anaesthetic to spread over
the mucosa. Only small doses of lignocaine are used but, never-
theless, systemic toxic effects may occur, and although they are rare
they may be serious in susceptible persons. Central nervous stimulation, confusion, delirium and convulsions may occur. This reaction is corrected by administering an injection of a short-acting
barbiturate such as amylobarbitone. Sudden respiratory and circulatory collapse may also occur and prove fatal. This procedure is
done about an hour before the operation is due. Normal premedication and immediate preparations should be carried out and the
patient left to rest quietly until it is time for his operation.

Post-operative care

On return from theatre the patient should be placed in the sitting
position, well supported by pillows, as soon as he is able. If the nose
is packed, the patient's respiratory function should be closely
observed so that any problems can be quickly dealt with.

There are four main problems the patient experiences following
nasal surgery:

(a) *Bleeding.* Because of the rich blood supply to the nasal mucosa,
bleeding or the oozing of serum can be troublesome.

(b) *Oedema.* The mucosa is very likely to become swollen due to
manipulation during surgery.

(c) *Watery discharge.* Irritation of the mucosa results in a vast
outpouring of secretion and hence a continuously 'running' nose.
A 'nose bag' will mop up these secretions and add to patient
comfort.

(d) *Pain and tenderness.* This can be quite marked as the nose has
a very good nerve supply.

Nasal packs

If packs have been inserted during the operation, these are usually removed the day after the operation or certainly by the second post-operative day. There is usually slight bleeding or a blood-stained serous discharge when the packs are removed. Any packs should be removed gently, and if any resistance is encountered the doctor should be informed so that he can assess the situation.

Decongestants

To help reduce the oedema steam inhalations with a few drops of tincture of benzoin compound (Friars balsam) or a few crystals of menthol are given three times daily for a few days.

Nose drops containing a decongestant (Table 2.2) may also be prescribed. When drops are being instilled into the nose, the patient should be lying down with his head back and slightly to one side. The head is then moved to the other side to allow drops to be instilled into the other nostril. This procedure ensures that the drops flow over the irregular surfaces of the nasal cavity and reach back to the nasopharynx. The patient should spit out any excess medication which flows into the pharynx. The dose must never be exceeded and this point should be emphasised to patients who are to instil their own medication on discharge.

Oral hygiene

Because of the need to mouth breathe, the mucous membranes of the mouth and pharynx become dry and uncomfortable. A good fluid intake and attention to oral hygiene is vital. Also, of course, the dried mucous membranes predispose to infection which may easily spread to the middle ear, salivary glands or lower respiratory tract.

Pain

Pain relief can usually be achieved by paracetamol or some similar analgesic, though some patients may need something stronger initially. To ensure a good night's sleep a sedative such as nitrazepam may be prescribed. Rest and relief from anxiety help to speed recovery. Keeping the patient informed of what is happening and good pre-operative preparation are other essential aspects of relieving anxiety.

It adds considerably to patient comfort if an even temperature and humidity can be maintained. Smoking or being in a smoky atmosphere is asking for trouble.

Observations

The temperature, pulse and respirations are recorded four hourly over the first 24 to 48 hours, and if these are normal and no complications have developed the patient can be prepared for discharge.

In caring for a patient with a fracture of the nose, it is as well to remember that there may be central nervous system involvement. It is, therefore, essential that neurological observations to assess conscious levels are carried out half hourly. The nurse should also observe and enquire of any watery nasal discharge. The patient may notice this particularly when he coughs or when defaecating and straining against a closed epiglottis as this raises intracranial pressure. If such a discharge is observed it should be tested for sugar using a Clinistix. If the test is positive, this may indicate cerebrospinal fluid rhinorrhoea, suggesting a fracture of the anterior fossa and a tear in the dura mater. Patients with this type of injury will require the services of a neurosurgeon.

Preparation for discharge

Before discharge, the doctor will ensure that there are no adhesions present between the septum and the turbinates and that there are no haematomas. Any adhesions are broken down while haematomas require to be aspirated.

If antibiotics are being given, the patient must get a supply to complete the course. He should be advised to avoid extremes of temperature and dry dusty atmospheres for two to three weeks. He should also keep away from large confined crowds to lessen the risk of infection.

The details of post-operative care described above apply equally to most patients following nasal surgery. The nurse must plan the nursing care after a careful assessment of the patient. Potential and actual problems can then be identified, so allowing for rational person-centred care. Frequent evaluation of care will ensure updating and modification of care plans according to need.

Three

The oral cavity, pharynx and larynx

THE ORAL CAVITY AND PHARYNX

Applied anatomy and physiology

The oral cavity

Most of the important anatomical features of the mouth can be easily seen (Fig. 3.1a, b). The inner surface of the upper and lower lips, the mucosal lining of the cheeks, the hard palate and floor of the mouth enclose the cavity. The mucosal lining is non-keratinising stratified squamous epithelium.

The anterior two thirds of the tongue has a rough dorsal surface covered by tiny papillae and demarcated posteriorly by the vallate papillae. The tongue's inferior surface is smooth, as is the floor of the mouth; two submandibular ducts open into the latter.

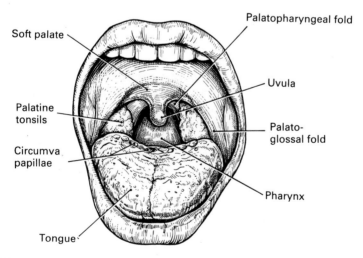

Fig. 3.1a Normal structure of mouth.

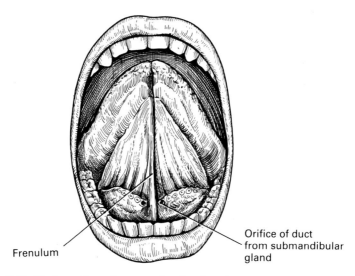

Frenulum

Orifice of duct
from submandibular
gland

Fig. 3.1b Undersurface of tongue showing frenulum.

The upper and lower alveoli separate the main body of the oral cavity from the buccal sulci. The parotid ducts open into the upper sulci at the level of the upper second molar teeth. There are two paired salivary glands: the parotid lies behind the vertical ramus of the mandible, while the submandibular glands lie inferior to its horizontal ramus. The sublingual gland lies below the tongue (Fig. 3.2).

Nasopharynx

'This area is bounded anteriorly by the choana and nasal septum and laterally by the Eustachian tubes and fossa of Rosenmuller; the floor is bounded by the soft palate. The roof is formed by the body of the sphenoid bone and is occupied by the adenoid pad in children (Fig. 2.1). The relationship between the adenoids and the Eustachian tube openings is of primary importance in middle ear disease.

During speech and swallowing the soft palate rises to close off the nasopharynx and, therefore, prevents food and liquid running along the nasal cavity.

Oropharynx

This area extends from the level of the hard palate above to the level of the hyoid bone below. Its anterior wall is regarded as the

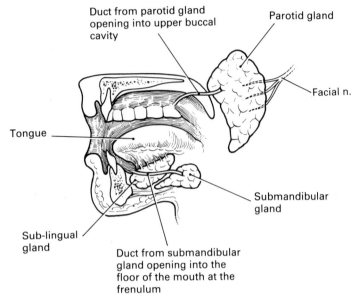

Duct from parotid gland opening into upper buccal cavity

Parotid gland

Facial n.

Tongue

Submandibular gland

Sub-lingual gland

Duct from submandibular gland opening into the floor of the mouth at the frenulum

Fig. 3.2 Salivary glands.

posterior third of the tongue (behind the vallate papillae and the anterior surface of the epiglottis). The lateral walls contain the tonsils lying in their fossae between the anterior and posterior tonsillar pillars (Fig. 3.1). The roof is the inferior surface of the soft palate and uvula. The area is again lined with squamous epithelium, and lymphoid tissue abounds, particularly in the tonsils and posterior third of the tongue.

The hypopharynx

This extends from the level of the hyoid and has three important anatomical areas; the posterior pharyngeal wall, the post-cricoid space and the pyriform fossae. These areas may be the site of tumours, which develop insidiously and are notoriously difficult to treat effectively.

Physiology of the oral cavity

The oral cavity is the first part of the gastro-intestinal tract. Food taken into the mouth is prepared here for swallowing, and early digestion of mainly cooked starches occurs. These are acted upon by ptyalin, an enzyme found in saliva. Saliva is secreted by the salivary glands. Once the food is thoroughly chewed and mixed with saliva, it is formed into a bolus which is propelled backwards by the tongue into the pharynx. The food is then propelled down into the oesophagus whilst, at the same time, the soft palate closes off the nasopharynx and the epiglottis closes the larynx.

Disorders of the oral cavity

Acute tonsillitis

Acute tonsillar infection (Fig. 3.3) is most common in young children; it is usually caused by a streptococcus. The condition is characterised by a sore throat, dysphagia, pyrexia and general malaise. There is often a referred otalgia. Examination reveals enlarged and tender cervical lymph nodes and acutely inflamed and enlarged tonsils.

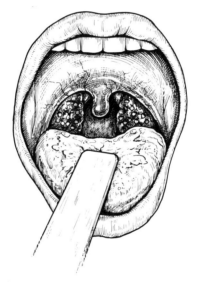

Fig. 3.3 Acute follicular tonsilitis.

Treatment and nursing care

Penicillin remains the treatment of choice as streptococcal infections are nearly always sensitive to this antibiotic. Bed rest is required whilst the patient is febrile. Soluble aspirin should be given in suitable dosage to relieve pain and discomfort. The patient should be encouraged to take sufficient fluids; 1 to 3 litres per day depending on age. Oral hygiene should be attended to regularly. When the patient is no longer febrile he should be allowed up but he should remain indoors. It is important that the course of penicillin be completed.

Complications

Acute otitis media is still a common accompaniment to acute. tonsillitis, as is the development of a peritonsillar abscess (Fig. 3.4). The renal and cardiac complications of streptococcal infection are less common now with adequate antibiotic cover.

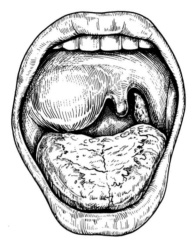

Fig. 3.4 Peritonsillar abscess. Abscess in peritonsillar space causing displacement of uvula.

Peritonsillar abscess (quinsy)

A quinsy is the collection of pus in the tissues outside the tonsillar capsule (Fig. 3.4). Tonsillitis in teenagers and young adults may spread to involve these tissues. This produces, initially, a peritonsillar cellulitis which progresses to abscess formation. Dysphagia worsens, pain becomes predominantly unilateral and the patient may be unable to open his mouth. This latter symptom, known as trismus, is the result of a spasm of the nearby pterygoid muscles.

Treatment and nursing care

Treatment, as for abscesses elsewhere, is by surgical drainage with antibiotic cover (Fig. 3.5). Parenteral antibiotics may be required

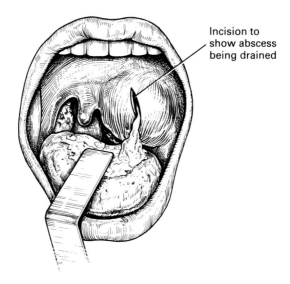

Incision to
show abscess
being drained

Fig. 3.5 Drainage of peritonsillar abscess.

along with intravenous fluids if dysphagia is severe. Medium-range analgesics will be required initially when the pain is severe. The nursing care is essentially the same as for acute tonsillitis with particular attention being paid to oral hygiene. A four-hourly temperature, pulse and respiration chart should be maintained until the condition has settled.

Tonsillectomy

Tonsillectomy is removal of the tonsils. There are many indications for this procedure:

(a) *Recurrent bouts of acute tonsillitis.* Each child must be assessed individually. Four or five attacks in one year with significant bouts of ill-health and loss of schooling are general factors which must be taken into account. It is important to establish that occasional symptoms of sore throat are in fact due to acute tonsillar infection and that the symptoms justify submitting a child to hospital admission and general anaesthesia for a procedure which is not without risk.

(b) *Previous peritonsillar abscess.* Tonsil removal is usually advocated following this condition. The operation is performed about six weeks after drainage of the abscess. This permanently removes the risk of recurrence.

(c) *Removal for histological examination.* This may be required if there is a suspicion of malignancy.

The operation

The operation is performed under a general anaesthetic. The most common procedure is dissection of the tonsils from their fossae, though in some places the guillotine method is still used in children.

Complications of tonsillectomy

(a) *Haemorrhage.* Dissection of the tonsils leaves a large raw area in the tonsillar fossa. Reactionary haemorrhage may occur within the first 24 hours of operation, and may be due to slippage of a ligature or elevation of blood pressure. In spite of careful monitoring of vital signs, blood loss may not be immediately apparent if blood is being swallowed. Once blood loss has been noted, however, the surgeon should be notified immediately. Delay in taking measures to control the problem is a recipe for disaster. Secondary haemorrhage may occur between the fifth and tenth day post-operatively and is related to sepsis in the tonsillar fossae. In general, it is a less serious problem. However, patients will usually be readmitted for observation until the problem settles.

(b) *Acute otitis media.* While referred earache is common following tonsillectomy, and self-limiting, acute middle ear infection may also occur.

Pre-operative care

Patients are generally admitted the day before surgery. A recent bout of acute tonsillitis or upper respiratory tract infection should be excluded to avoid problems of excessive blood loss and general anaesthesia. Even a vague suspicion of a bleeding tendency requires investigation prior to surgery. This can easily be established by blood coagulation studies.

The patient's mouth should be examined. A note should be made of loose teeth, particularly in children, and of dental crowns in adults, since the Boyle Davis gag used during operation may

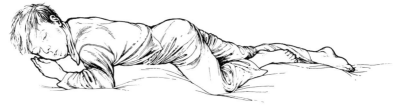

Fig. 3.6 Tonsillectomy position.

dislodge them. The danger is of aspiration of the loose tooth or crown into the bronchial tree. Loose primary teeth can easily be removed under general anaesthetic.

Post-operative care of the tonsillectomy patient demands a high degree of nursing skill and experience. On return to the ward the patient is placed in the semi-prone (tonsillectomy) position (Fig. 3.6), so that any blood or saliva will run out of the mouth. A check is made to ensure that the airway is clear. Recordings of pulse and blood pressure begin and are continued half-hourly. The nurse should observe that breathing is normal and note any excessive swallowing. Any suspicion of bleeding requires inspection of the mouth with a good light. If bleeding occurs, a cold compress may be applied to the neck and side of the face while the surgeon is being informed.

Three to four hours post-operatively, the patient should have his hands and face washed and be changed into fresh nightclothes. A mouth wash is given and the patient is encouraged to drink. Jelly and ice cream are also offered at this time. This is soothing and helps to ease the pain and encourage early swallowing, which prevents the muscles tensing up. A good deal of persuasion may be needed, but if the patient persists, swallowing will soon become easier. Failure to eat and swallow may result in infection of the tonsil bed. Paracetamol elixir adequately provides pain relief in children. Aspirin mixture, which was used in the past, may increase the tendency to bleed as a result of its anti-platelet activity. Adults may require pethidine or a similar strength of analgesia post-operatively. Referred otalgia is common, but the ears should be examined to ensure that an acute otitis media is not missed.

Post-operative progress is rapid, with swallowing virtually back to normal within forty-eight hours. Bed rest is preferable for the first 24 hours, but the patient is allowed up to the toilet on the evening of the operation. However, the after-effects of general anaesthesia and blood loss may cause some faintness, so the patient should not be left alone while he is up.

Discharge from hospital is variable, some patients being fit for discharge on the first or second post-operative day. Children from deprived homes should be detained longer. The child's parents should be informed of the possibility of bleeding and given instructions to return to hospital if it is persistent. A greyish slough grows over the operation site. This is quite normal and parents should be reassured that it will soon clear. Good oral hygiene is essential. The child should be kept off school for about two weeks and should avoid extremes of temperature and crowded public places. Similar general rules also relate to adults.

Oral hygiene measures

Following radiotherapy to the head and neck and treatment by cytotoxic drugs, oral discomfort is often a problem. Pain, inability to chew, difficulty in opening the mouth, xerostomia (dry mouth) and mucositis are the most common changes. In addition, the lateral borders of the tongue become denuded, and a pseudomembrane forms, which eventually peels off. The saliva which is produced consolidates into mucus and viscous matter. All of this combines to make chewing, swallowing and speech difficult. Cytotoxic drugs and the effects of the cancer weaken the bodies' immune defence mechanisms so that secondary infection, often of fungal or viral origin, can also be a problem. Some drugs in particular cause local and diffuse oral lesions which make normal hygiene measures painful. Gingivitis and bleeding from the gums may also occur, especially if platelet counts are low. The pain and discomfort and apparent complexity of the problem may tempt nurses to stop all oral hygiene measures. This is a great mistake, as much can and should be done. Firstly, the patient can be reassured that on completion of the treatment the disturbed oral function will quickly recover. Those patients who are able should clean their own mouths, using a soft toothbrush which will not further damage the mucous membranes. A high fluid intake is encouraged and frequent non-acidic mouth washes should be given. Artificial salivas containing substances such as carboxymethylcellulose, sorbitol and minerals are useful. They have two main actions: firstly, they are lubricants, and secondly, they buffer the acidity of the mouth. Where there is a superimposed infection, frequent mouth washes with solutions of sodium bicarbonate will help to cleanse the tissues. The solution will also reduce pain and discomfort by relieving some of the dryness. In the case of fungal infections, an anti-fungicidal drug such as Nystatin can be applied locally in the mouth. No attempt should be made to scrape off fungal patches as this causes bleeding and makes the mouth condition worse. When assessing oral hygiene needs, always use a good light and make a thorough inspection of all the buccal surfaces, tongue and teeth. If there appear to be dental problems, the doctor will arrange for a dental surgeon to see the patient. He will treat and advise. This is very important before radiotherapy or cytotherapy treatment begins. Both forms of therapy lead to a degree of immunosuppression and, therefore, dental caries could be a ready focus of infection. There is also the risk of radiation necrosis of the mandible in patients with dental caries.

The adenoids

The adenoid pad of lymphoid tissue lies in the nasopharynx (Fig. 2.1). It is large in children, gradually becoming smaller in size during the early teens. Like the tonsils it may become the focus of recurrent infection, and may be removed at the same time as the tonsils in adenotonsillectomy.

Infection causes the adenoid pad to enlarge. This results in blockage of the lower end of the Eustachian tube and is associated with the development of secretory otitis media (p. 17). Mouthbreathing and snoring may also occur, indicating partial obstruction to normal nasal respiration.

Removal is achieved by use of an adenoid curette, which effectively scrapes the lymphoid tissue out of the nasopharynx. Occasionally, primary haemorrhage requires the insertion of a postnasal pack (Fig. 2.12). In the main, however, it causes less upset to the child than tonsillectomy.

Neoplasm of the oral cavity and pharynx

Squamous carcinoma is the commonest type of cancer in this area. A complaint of an ulcer of the tongue or buccal mucosa may be the first indication, while tumours in the oro- and hypopharynx present with discomfort or difficulty in swallowing. Lymphomas may develop at the sites of lymphoid tissue in the tongue base and tonsils.

In general, the treatment of choice for such neoplasm is radiotherapy. The results depend upon tumour site, size and spread: those in the pyriform fossae and post-cricoid regions have a particularly poor outlook. (See the section on 'Oral hygiene measures' for the special oral hygiene measures required.) Tumours in this region are very distressing and uncomfortable; they make eating, drinking and communication difficult. It is important to ensure that the patient receives adequate food and fluids. A fluid balance chart and regular weighing are essential. Analgesics for pain relief should be given, following the assessment of individual need. The patient's relatives also need support at this time and should, whenever possible, be involved in the care of the patient.

Foreign bodies in the pharynx and oesophagus

Swallowed fish bones may become stuck in the tongue base or tonsils, causing discomfort on swallowing. Usually, they are easily seen and removed. Young children may swallow coins or small toys while playing. Adults, particularly those with dentures, may fail to chew meat properly and as a result it becomes lodged in the oesophagus (Fig. 3.7). Meat or chicken bones may also be swallowed. Deliberate swallowing of dangerous objects is not uncommon among psychiatrically disturbed patients.

There are three sites at which obstruction occurs: at the cricopharyngeal sphincter, at the cardiac sphincter and at a point midway between them where the aorta compresses the oesophagus.

Complete obstruction results in the patient being unable to swallow his saliva. For most foreign bodies the patient is able to localise the site of obstruction.

The major risk is of perforation of the pharynx or oesophagus, especially with impacted bones, safety pins or other sharp objects. Oesophagoscopy and removal of the foreign body under general anaesthesia is required.

The patient should be nursed in the upright position. Observation of pulse, respirations and blood pressure should be recorded half hourly, or more frequently, depending on the nature of the foreign body and level of obstruction. The patient should have strictly nil by mouth, and a basin should be provided to enable him to spit out saliva. Any increase in pain or discomfort should be reported to the surgeon. Preparation is as for any operation under general anaesthetic. Time must be allowed for the stomach to empty if food or fluids have been taken. The doctor must get consent for the procedure.

Oesophagoscopy and pharyngoscopy

Direct examination of the pharynx and oesophagus is performed frequently for both diagnostic reasons and for the

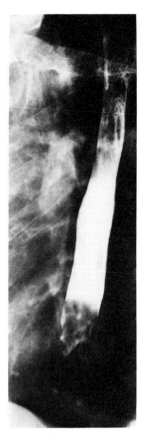

Fig. 3.7 Foreign body in oesophagus.

removal of foreign bodies. While rigid endoscopes are required for the removal of foreign bodies, flexible endoscopes are also in common use.

Good post-operative care of these patients is essential to ensure that perforation, etc. will be diagnosed early. Patients with pharyngeal or oesophageal carcinomas or strictures are at particular risk.

Pharyngeal perforation. Local pain in the neck and on swallowing saliva is the first complaint. The leakage of saliva and air occurs into the soft tissues of the neck, the latter causing surgical emphysema.

Oesophageal perforation is characterised by pain in the back, between the scapula, and by a rising pulse and pyrexia. Leakage into the tissues of the mediastinum is a serious condition.

Following examination, T.P.R. recordings are made. No oral fluids are allowed for the first few hours until the patient is completely awake following anaesthesia. Oral fluids are gradually introduced, and any symptoms of perforation should be reported to the surgeon immediately.

Dysphagia

This can be described as difficulty in swallowing. However, it is a symptom which requires full and thorough investigation. There are many causes for it.

(a) Painful conditions of the mouth or oropharynx, such as aphthous ulceration or tonsillitis, may make swallowing uncomfortable. There will be no history of obstruction to swallowing and the cause will be readily apparent.

(b) Many patients complain of a 'lump in the throat'. This strange sensation is often associated with the reflux of gastric secretion found with hiatus hernia. Any doubt as to the exact cause, however, requires direct examination under anaesthetic of the pharynx and oesophagus.

(c) *Oesophageal strictures.* Narrowing of the lower third of the oesophagus is often a result of the longstanding reflux oesophagitis associated with hiatus hernia. Diagnosis is made by barium swallow and meal and by oesophagoscopy. Severe symptoms of dysphagia may require that the stricture be dilated. This procedure is not without risk of oesophageal perforation.

(d) *Carcinoma of the pharynx.* The post-cricoid region and the pyriform fossae are sites of involvement. In general, dysphagia is a late symptom presenting when the tumour is large. Some patients may only present when spread to cervical lymph nodes becomes apparent. Treatment is usually by radiotherapy. If surgical removal of the pharynx is undertaken, then it is replaced either by a segment of colon or stomach brought up through the chest, or by raising a flap of skin from the chest wall to fashion into a tube-like structure. Both procedures represent major surgical problems. Overall, the outlook is poor, irrespective of treatment offered.

(e) *Carcinoma of the oesophagus.* Progressive dysphagia and weight loss are the sinister symptoms of this condition. Treatment is by surgery or radiotherapy. As with pharyngeal tumours, the morbidity associated with treatment is high and overall results are poor.

THE LARYNX
Applied anatomy and physiology

The structure of the larynx is based on a cartilaginous skeleton (Fig. 3.8) which provides protection for its internal components. The thyroid cartilage consists of two broad plates which join to form the apex or Adam's apple. It sits above and articulates with the cricoid cartilage, which forms a complete ring around the upper end of the trachea. Two arytenoid cartilages articulate with the upper border of the posterior part of the cricoid. These are pyramidal in shape, and a fibrous band is attached to their anterior processes which runs to the apex of the thyroid cartilage to form the vocal cord.

The mobile epiglottis is a leaf-shaped cartilage, attached just above the vocal cords at the apex of the thyroid cartilage. Folds of mucosa, known as the ary-epiglottic folds, run from it to the arytenoid cartilages on each side.

The movements of these various components of the larynx are complex and are controlled by several groups of muscles, both within and outside the laryngeal skeleton. Their nerve supply is from the recurrent laryngeal nerve, a vagal branch which lies in the groove between the trachea and oesophagus. This nerve is particularly vulnerable to damage, especially during surgery of the thyroid gland. On the left side, the recurrent laryngeal nerve takes a long course into the chest before doubling back to supply the larynx. It can be damaged by the spread of bronchial carcinoma and during certain types of cardiac surgery.

The mucosa of the larynx is stratified squamous epithelium. The larynx has two important physiological functions:

(a) *Airway protection*. During swallowing or vomiting the epiglottis falls backwards to seal off the larynx. In addition, three laryngeal sphincters operate. The ary-epiglottic folds come together as do the false and true cords.

Should food particles reach the larynx, stimulation of the very senstive mucosal lining produces a rapid cough reflex.

(b) *Phonation*. During quiet respiration the vocal cords separate in abduction. During speech the cords come together in adduction, and vibrations set up by the passage of air from below are articulated by the mouth and tongue to form speech.

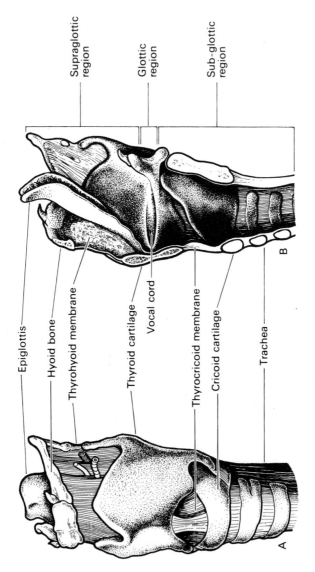

Fig. 3.8 Larynx. A. Front view. B. Saggital view.

Tracheostomy

This important operation creates an artificial opening in the anterior tracheal wall just below the cricoid cartilage (Figs. 3.9 and 3.10). A plastic or metal tube can then be inserted to maintain its patency.

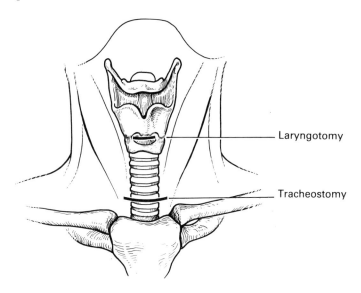

Laryngotomy

Tracheostomy

Fig. 3.9 Incisions for elective laryngotomy and tracheostomy.

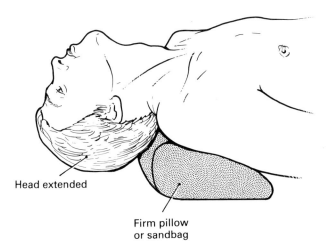

Head extended

Firm pillow
or sandbag

Fig. 3.10 Position of patient for tracheostomy.

Use of this procedure is not confined to ENT patients, since it has a place in the management of a wide variety of surgical and medical problems. There are several broad indications for it:

(a) *Relief of upper airways obstruction.* Trauma, acute infection such as epiglottitis, foreign bodies and advanced laryngeal tumours are some examples of conditions which may block off the larynx, producing stridor. Tracheostomy under these circumstances may prove to be life-saving.

(b) *Protection of the bronchial tree.* Under normal circumstances, the larynx prevents inhalation of food, saliva or vomit. This protective effect is absent in patients in deep coma as a result of head injury or drug overdose. A tracheostomy tube with an inflatable cuff will seal off the lower respiratory tract in these circumstances (Fig. 3.8a).

(c) *Respiratory insufficiency.* Patients with severe pneumonia or multiple fractured ribs may be unable to ventilate their lungs sufficiently well to maintain normal blood gas levels. Tracheostomy has several advantages: it allows easier removal of bronchial secretions by suction, and also reduces the amount of so-called dead space, since the patient no longer has to expend effort to shift air through the upper airways.

(d) *Long-term ventilation.* If for any reason this is required, then a tracheostomy tube is preferable to an endotracheal tube, since the latter type will eventually damage the mucosal lining of the larynx if it is left in place too long.

Tracheostomy tubes

These may be either metal or plastic (Figs. 3.11a and 3.11b).

(a) *Silver tubes.* This type may be single or designed with an outer tube—this remains in position in the tracheostomy stoma while the inner tube can be removed for cleaning. Some tubes may have a valve mechanisms which allows normal speech.

(b) *Disposable plastic tubes* are in common use. They may be plain or designed with an inflatable balloon cuff which can be used to seal off the trachea for positive pressure ventilation. This will prevent anaesthetic gases from leaking back alongside the tube.

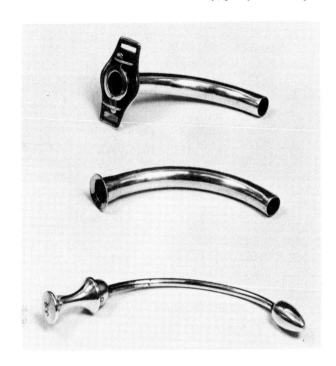

A

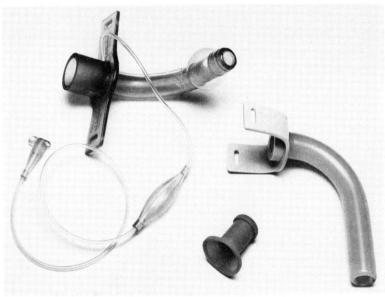

B

Fig. 3.11 (a) Silver tracheostomy tube. (b) Cuffed tracheostomy tube, plain tracheostomy tube, stoma button.

The complications of tracheostomy

(a) *Tube dislodgement*. The tracheostomy tube should be secured by tapes around the patient's neck; it may also be sutured to the patient's skin. The wound edges should be held apart by tracheal dilators until a clean tube is inserted.

(b) *Tube obstruction*. Inspissated bronchial secretion may cause this. If the tube is not cleared by suction then the doctor should be informed. The tube may require to be removed and an attempt made to clear the obstruction with forceps. Occasionally, a flexible bronchoscope may be required to search for and remove the obstructing plug of mucus.

(c) *Surgical emphysema*. Air escapes into the soft tissues of the neck, producing a characteristic crackling sensation on palpation. Small amounts of air are of little significance. Large quantities, however, may cause respiratory embarrassment. Emphysema will develop if the tracheostomy wound is sutured too tightly.

(d) *Haemorrhage*. A partially dislodged tube may lie at an abnormal angle and erode the anterior tracheal wall. Erosion of the innominate artery may result in fatal bleeding.

(e) *Pneumonia*. This is an ever present risk in all tracheostomy patients. Strictly aseptic procedures and adequate chest physiotherapy will avoid this problem.

(f) *Tracheo-oesophageal fistula*. This may develop if an over-inflated cuff is allowed to cause pressure necrosis of the posterior tracheal wall. Saliva and food are then liable to trickle into the bronchial tree producing severe aspiration pneumonia.

(g) *Decannulation*. The long-term tracheostomy patient becomes used to his new situation, and sudden removal of the tracheostomy tube may cause respiratory distress. Partial and gradual blocking-off is required, usually by means of corks cut to size, until finally the tube is completely blocked off for 24 hours. It will then be safe to remove the tracheostomy tube. Decannulation is a particularly difficult problem in children.

Post-operative care of the tracheostomy

An appreciation of the potential complications of the procedure is essential for the intelligent care of these patients. On return from theatre the patient should be placed in an upright position, well supported by pillows. A check should be made to ensure that the tracheostomy tube is securely in place, in the correct position and free of all obstruction. T.P.R. and blood pressure recordings should begin.

Communication

The patient should not be left alone for the first 24–48 hours postoperatively, and provision should be made for him to communicate either by means of a note-pad and pencil or by a magic slate. A spare tracheostomy tube of the correct size along with sterile tracheal dilators should be close at hand.

Tracheostomy tube

A cuffed tube (Fig. 3.11b) will have been inserted by the surgeon, and cuff inflation can be maintained for the first 24 hours or longer if positive pressure ventilation is used. Pressure necrosis of the tracheal mucosa is avoided if the cuff is deflated for 5 minutes in every hour. Re-inflation of the cuff to the correct amount can be achieved in patients who are being ventilated. This is done by the 'minimal leak technique', whereby the cuff is inflated only to a volume which will allow a minimal leak to escape.

Suction

In the immediate post-operative period, frequent suction will be required to prevent the accumulation of bronchial secretions. Inspired air is no longer humidified by the nasal mucosa so that himidification must be provided to prevent drying of the bronchial mucosa. This will aid suction removal. Clearing of secretions helps to prevent paroxysms of coughing which may be very distressing for the patient. Patients will vary in the quantity of secretion they produce, so that a strict regime should not be applied to every patient. Those with a history of chronic obstructive airways disease and bronchitis will obviously require a more frequent bronchial toilet.

A strict aseptic technique is required when suction equipment is used, and a gown and mask should be worn. A sterile suction catheter is used, which should have a diameter not greater than half that of the tracheostomy tube. Careful explanation to the patient is necessary. The hands are washed and dried and the catheter pack opened. The catheter is then inserted into one limb of the Y-connection which has been previously inserted into the suction tubing. Suction pressure is adjusted to be not more than 600 mmHg. The hands are washed again and sterile gloves put on. The suction tubing is picked up at the Y-connection, allowing the protective wrapping of the catheter to fall off. Using the gloved hand (or sterile forceps), the tip of the catheter is inserted into the tracheal lumen for 10–15 cm. Once in position, the open limb of the Y-connection is occluded with the thumb to apply suction, while the catheter is slowly withdrawn and rotated. Only short periods of suction, lasting a few seconds, should be carried out. If secretions prove thick and tenacious, 5 ml of sterile saline can be injected into the trachea to liquefy secretions and permit easier suction. When the procedure is completed, the suction tubing should be flushed out and the catheter discarded. Co-operation with the physiotherapist will allow deeply seated secretions to be mobilised. If a specimen is required for bacteriological culture and a suitable specimen of secretion cannot be obtained, the catheter tip can be cut off and cultured.

Repeated bouts of suction can be very tiring for patients. Nursing care must be planned carefully to ensure that the patient is not exhausted by it.

Tracheostomy tubes, once inserted, are left for a period of 4–5 days before they are changed for the first time. This procedure should be performed preferably by the surgeon responsible for the tracheostomy.

Removal of tracheostomy tube

In many patients the tracheostomy will not be a permanent need. In these circumstances, it should be removed as soon as it is practical to do so. Many patients will require to be 'weaned off' the tracheostomy tube. They have to relearn to breathe through their nose once more and may find this very difficult. To overcome this the tracheostomy tube should be closed off for increasing periods of time until the patient can breathe normally once more. Once the tube has been removed, a dry dressing is applied and within a few days the stoma will shrink and heal over. In some patients, especially children, closure may have to be facilitated by the surgeon. Only very minimal scarring should be evident in the long term and patients should be reassured of this.

Disorders of the larynx

Acute laryngitis

This common condition is associated with upper respiratory tract infection, usually viral in origin. Hoarseness, or even complete loss of voice, may occur in association with pain in the throat. Voice rest is important to ensure that the hoarseness resolves, and smoking should be discouraged. In most patients, complete recovery can be expected. However, the condition may become chronic, with persisting hoarseness. Such cases require full examination to exclude more sinister causes of hoarseness.

Vocal cord polyps

Localised oedema of the vocal cords may result in polyp formation (Fig. 3.12). The aetiological factors are similar to acute laryngitis, with voice abuse as a major factor. Effective treatment may require surgical removal. Again, however, voice rest is important for a complete recovery.

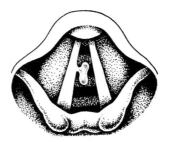

Fig. 3.12 Polyps of vocal cord.

Vocal cord nodules

These small fibrous nodules develop at the junction of the anterior and middle thirds of the vocal cords. They vary greatly in size and tend to affect people who over-use their voice, such as school teachers and amateur singers. Resolution of small nodules may be achieved by appropriate speech therapy. Large nodules require surgical removal. It is interesting that children also develop this lesion, when it is descriptively termed 'screamer's nodules'.

Tumours of the larynx

These may be benign or malignant. The majority of the latter are squamous carcinomas and they are classified according to site, arising in the supraglottis (above the vocal cords), the subglottis (below the cords), and the glottis (involving the vocal cords themselves) (Fig. 3.13a, b and c).

Tumours of the vocal cords are most common, presenting early with hoarseness. Supra- and subglottic tumours tend to present later. While there are many possible causes of hoarseness, most of which are benign, the possibility of malignant disease must always be considered.

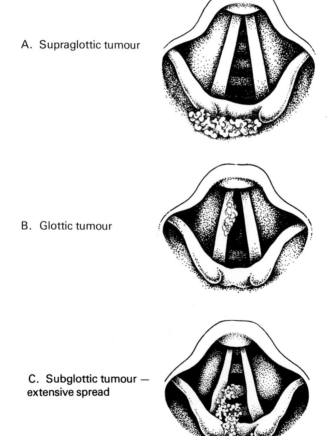

A. Supraglottic tumour

B. Glottic tumour

C. Subglottic tumour — extensive spread

Fig. 3.13 (a,b,c) Tumours of the larynx.

General practitioners will always refer patients whose symptoms fail to improve satisfactorily within two or three weeks for full investigation.

In the management of tumours of the larynx there are two major considerations. Obviously, the first aim of treatment is to completely eradicate disease: the second aim is, to preserve normal function of the larynx, if possible, since the loss of a normal voice is a devastating blow, affecting all aspects of the patient's lifestyle. Radiotherapy is, therefore, offered to the majority of patients in the first instance, and the outlook for small tumours diagnosed early is excellent.

Large tumours, or those which have spread to cervical lymph nodes, require surgical treatment, with removal of the larynx along with the affected lymph nodes if necessary (Fig. 3.14).

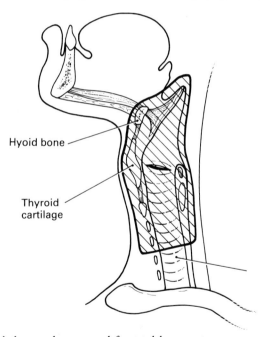

Hyoid bone

Thyroid cartilage

Fig. 3.14 Area to be removed for total laryngectomy.

Laryngectomy

If the larynx is removed, the cut end of the trachea must be fashioned to form a permanent tracheostomy opening (Figs. 3.15 and 3.16). A team approach is necessary for the care of such patients, as will be outlined below.

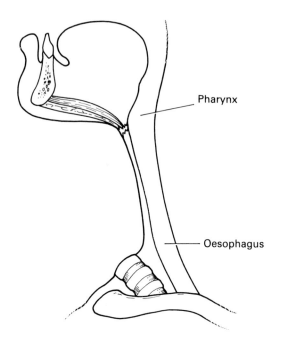

Fig. 3.15 Position of tracheal opening on completion of total laryngectomy.

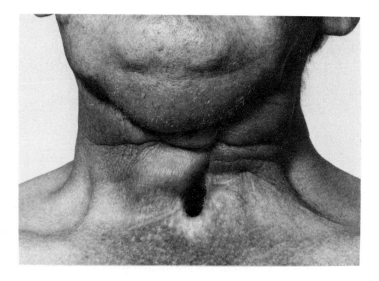

Fig. 3.16 Permanent tracheostomy stoma.

Pre-operative care

The patient will be admitted several days prior to surgery, since careful pre-operative care will certainly ensure a smooth post-operative period. It is the surgeon's responsibility to explain the nature of the proposed operation, both with the patient and with supportive relatives. His general condition will be assessed, with special attention being paid to the state of dentition and nutrition. Many patients are heavy smokers and will require chest physiotherapy before as well as after surgery. Because speech rehabilitation forms such a large part of the care of laryngectomy patients, the speech therapists will also see him. They will also arrange for a patient who has previously undergone the operation and subsequently achieved good voice production, to meet the patient, if the patient would like this. Much useful information is exchanged during such meetings which are usually very effective for boosting morale.

The patient is prepared as for any major surgery. The patient should be told which part of the ward he will be nursed in. If possible, the same nurses who prepare him for surgery should care for him after the operation. The need for an intravenous infusion and nasogastric tube should be explained. The face and upper chest of the patient, if male, should be shaved on the morning of the operation. Breathing exercises are very important following the operation, and these should be taught before the operation. The physiotherapist will help with this.

Post-operative care

The patient should be nursed in the sitting position and care of the tracheostomy commences as outlined previously. Recording of vital signs is important.

Because the pharynx is reconstructed following the removal of the larynx, the patient will be fed by a nasogastric tube for several days following surgery. Proprietary nasogastric feeding preparations are convenient to use and ensure that adequate nutrition is provided.

The surgeon will advise when oral fluids can be introduced. Over a few days the patient will progress to semi-solids, then to solids. A fluid balance chart is essential. Initially, the patient will not even be able to swallow his saliva and suction will necessary. The patient can no longer clear his nostrils, so that these also should be cleaned. If crusting is a problem, dressed orange sticks soaked in a sodium bicarbonate solution can be used. The nostrils can then be lightly smeared with Vaseline. Suction catheters, used to remove oral and nasal secretions, must never be used to clear secretions from the tracheostomy.

The patient should be mobilised as soon as he is able. Most patients will be able to get up the first or second post-operative day. If fluids are well tolerated via the nasogastric tube, the intravenous infusion can be discontinued, so that getting the patient up and mobilised becomes easier.

Wound drains

Because skin flaps are raised during the operation, suction drains are placed beneath them at the end of the operation. This is to ensure that no blood or serous fluid collects below them, since this would be detrimental to wound healing. Checks should, therefore, be made regularly to ensure that suction drains are functioning properly at all times.

The suction drains are removed in 48 to 72 hours, whilst sutures are removed in seven to ten days. Fistula can sometimes be a problem, and oral feeding may have to be delayed until they heal. Initially, the patient will usually have a cuffed tracheostomy tube, progressing later to a silver tube (Fig. 3.11a) or stoma button (Fig. 3.11b).

Bowel management

Constipation may be a problem as the patient is no longer able to perform the Valsalva manoeuvre. The introduction of bulking agents and fibre to the diet will help. Initially suppositories or an enema may be required. Flatulence and/or diarrhoea can also occur with tube feeding, which is very distressing for patients who are recovering from a major operation. Care in administering the tube feeds and the use of a flatus tube and/or a carminative, such as peppermint water, will usually give relief. If diarrhoea persists, the tube feed should be changed to half strength for a day or two or switched to another brand of feed.

Communication

Communication by means of a note-pad and pencil is essential and patience shown by both nursing and medical staff will prevent the patient becoming frustrated.

Speech therapy begins as soon as the nasogastric tube is removed. The patient is encouraged to swallow air into the pharynx and oesophagus, and is taught to belch the air. This can then be used to form words by the mouth, lips and tongue. This oesophageal speech is very effective. However, not all patients achieve it, since a high degree of motivation is required for a successful outcome. There are various mechanical devices available to aid speech if this is not attained.

Stoma care

Much time should be spent by the nurses in preparing the patient to manage the stoma on his own. Initially, secretions will have to be aspirated and this may be necessary morning and evening during the first few months following the operation. The need for this will decline over time and will only usually be a problem if the patient has a chest infection. Small portable suction pumps are available and most patients or a relative will soon learn how to use them effectively. Humidification and protection of the stoma can be achieved by the use of one of the various 'stoma aprons' available for this purpose. These cover the stoma and are secured by tapes around the neck. They prevent dust etc. from entering the bronchial tree. Most patients prefer to have the stoma covered and are usually quite ingenious at making the stoma quite unobtrusive. Patients must take great care not to let water into the stoma when bathing. There are devices on the market for use when the patient is swimming, though these need careful fitting by the surgeon. There is no reason why the patient should not enjoy a full life provided he is sensible and prudent in his daily living activities.

Stridor

Obstruction to normal respiration produces this symptom; it demands early and effective treatment, particularly in children. There are several causes for it.

(a) *Inhaled foreign bodies.* This is a common occurrence in children, frequently caused by peanuts or sweets. As the object enters the larynx there is explosive coughing with stridor, and if total obstruction occurs the child may become cyanosed. Often it passes on into the trachea or right main bronchus and the child recovers. The history, however, indicates that foreign body aspiration has occurred, and that bronchoscopy is required for its removal.

(b) *Acute epiglottitis*. This infection is caused by the Haemophilus organism, producing marked oedema of the epiglottis and respiratory obstruction. The history of stridor is short. Admission to hospital will allow prompt examination of the child under anaesthesia and the insertion of an endotracheal or nasotracheal tube. Tracheostomy may be required. Treatment with antibiotics and steroids will allow the swelling to resolve.

(c) *Congenital stridor*. The symptom may be apparent at birth and will gradually improve as the child grows. Common causes are laryngeal webs lying between the vocal cords, or rarely, congenital tumours or cysts.

(d) *Laryngeal tumours*. Both benign and malignant tumours may cause stridor.

Vocal cord palsy

Weakness of the vocal cords results from any condition which damages the nerve supply to the larynx (Fig. 3.17). In general, weakness of one cord is not a great problem. Bilateral palsy is much more serious.

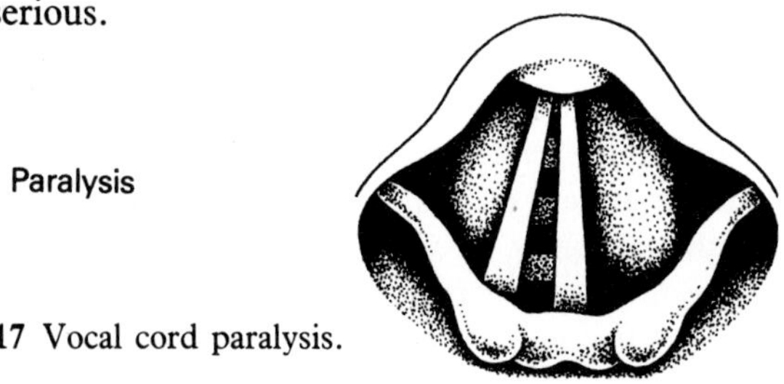

Paralysis

Fig. 3.17 Vocal cord paralysis.

Bilateral abductor palsy

This problem may arise if both recurrent laryngeal nerves are damaged by, for example, thyroid surgery. Failure of the vocal cords to separate results in respiratory obstruction and stridor. As a result, a permanent tracheostomy is required.

Bilateral adductor palsy

Failure of the vocal cords to close means that the lower respiratory tract is not protected from the inhalation of food and saliva. This state of affairs is serious and often ends with fatal aspiration pneumonia.

Appendix One
Hearing aids

Advances in technology over the past 20 years have led to the production of hearing aids which provide effective amplification for various degrees of handicap. Not only people with conductive type hearing loss but also those with sensorineural hearing loss benefit from a properly fitted hearing aid. Indeed all forms of hearing loss—conductive, sensorineural, unilateral, high frequency, severe hearing impairment, mild hearing loss- or even those with reduced tolerance to loud sounds can all benefit. It is essential to establish the cause of the hearing loss before hearing aids are fitted. Persons discovered to have a hearing loss should have a thorough assessment by an ENT specialist and treatable conditions should be treated. Thereafter the person will be referred to an Audiology/Hearing Aid Clinic for the testing and fitting of the most suitable hearing aid. Many people, especially the elderly, will deny they have any hearing loss whilst others may acknowledge the problem but refuse to wear a hearing aid. Often this is because they have not persevered long enough with the aid to get optimal use from it. They may complain that their greatest problem is in noisy places and that the aid makes the situation worse. It is essential when the hearing aid is supplied that the person is given realistic expectations of what the hearing aid will and will not do. The hearing aid specialist will help in the selection and orientation of a hearing aid which best suits the individual's needs.

The hearing aid is a small electronic device that serves as an aid to hearing. It will not solve all the patient's communication problems. What needs to be impressed on the user is that it will make all sounds louder including less desirable sounds. Whilst the normal ear can sort out sounds in a noisy room for example, the person using a hearing aid may have great difficulty in separating speech from background noise. This makes social interaction difficult and may lead the user to abandon his aid. With patience the majority of users will learn to get real benefit from their hearing aid.

Types of hearing aid

There are two types of hearing aid in common use: behind-the-ear hearing aids (BE), and body worn aids (BW) as shown in Figures 1.19 and 1.20. As mentioned above, hearing aids are designed to meet different degrees and types of hearing loss. The National Health Service provide both behind-the-ear and body worn aids. The post-aural hearing aids provided are the:

BE 10 Series—mild to moderate hearing loss
BE 30 Series—more than moderate hearing loss
BE 50 Series—profound hearing loss

The hearing aid has a small microphone which picks up sound and amplifies it. The amplified sound is delivered to the ear via a rigid curved acoustic elbow and plastic tubing which fits into the earmould. In some behind-the-ear hearing aids the microphone is forward facing (Fig. 1.19 top left hand corner). This arrangement is helpful to people who are at school or attending lectures.

The body worn aids are much larger and therefore more conspicuous. There are two aids of this type currently available from the N.H.S.

BW 61—mild to moderate hearing loss
BW 81—profound hearing loss

On body worn aids (Fig. 1.20 (a) and (b)) the earphone is connected to the aid by a flexible wire. The earphone fits into the earmould (Fig. 1.20).

All hearing aids have on ON/OFF switch and VOLUME control to adjust loudness. On some models the on/off switch and volume control are combined. In addition, most hearing aids have a small switch marked 'T' for use when using the telephone. To get use of this facility British Telecom have first to fit an 'inductive coupler' in the telephone handset. The hearing aid contains a tiny coil which reacts with the inductive coupler to give better clarity of incoming speech and elimination of background noise. People with normal hearing will not notice any difference when using the adapted handset. Many public telephones are now fitted with the inductive coupler. When using the telephone the user has to place the earpiece of the handset over the microphone in the aid. Many hearing aid users also benefit if 'induction loops' are fitted in public places such as cinemas and theatres.

The controls on body-worn aids are larger and hence easier to manipulate. Because of this, arthritic patients are usually fitted with the BW61 type aids.

In addition to the controls mentioned above both behind-the-ear and body-worn aids have other controls. Users are strongly advised not to touch these controls but to return the aid to the hearing aid clinic. Faulty setting of the hearing aid may cause damage to the ear.

Power for hearing aids

Hearing aids are powered by batteries. It is essential that the batteries are fitted properly. Figure 1.19 shows the battery compartment open and the battery in situ. Note the '+' on both the battery and the aid. It is important to fit only recommended batteries. Recently, long-acting air-activated alkaline batteries have been introduced. These, as the name implies, are activated by air. It is important not to remove the sealing tab until just before fitting a new battery. The BE50 series which provides high amplification requires special mercury batteries. The body-worn hearing aids are fitted with torch-type batteries which must also be appropriate to the hearing aid.

Ear moulds

All hearing aids are fitted with an ear mould. This part of the aid is custom made for the user. This ensures that it fits snugly into the ear and should not rub or cause irritation. The earphone should be fitted firmly to the earmould to prevent whistling. The earmould will require cleaning and for this it should be completely disconnected from the hearing aid. It can then be washed in warm, soapy water, rinsed and dried. If the tube is blocked it can be cleaned using a pipe cleaner. Any water remaining in the tube can be removed by blowing through it. It is important not to wet the hearing aid itself. In the behind-the-ear aids the flexible plastic tubing that connects it to the earmould needs to be changed every few months as it becomes hard, cracks or collapses.

Users of hearing aids are provided with a small handbook entitled, *General Guidance for Hearing Aid Users*. This booklet is published by the government and is free of charge.

Hearing aid clinics

Hearing aid clinics are staffed by people specially trained to provide a comprehensive service to the hearing aid user. Clinics are to be found in all large centres usually within a hospital out-patient department. In addition, clinic staff visit smaller outlying areas on a regular basis.

All hearing aids supplied by the N.H.S. are free. Batteries available from the main hearing aid clinic and most local health clinics are also free of charge. Like any complex piece of equipment the hearing aid will require repair and maintenance and this is also free of charge. The hearing aid can either be brought to the clinic or sent by post. The user must produce his record book when repairs or batteries are required.

Follow-up care and education

Many different professionals are available to help the person with hearing loss; these include teachers for the deaf, peripatetic teachers, speech therapists and child psychologists. In addition, many other organisations will provide help and information for hearing aid users, in particular, The Royal National Institute for the Deaf.

The quality of life of anyone experiencing a hearing loss can be considerably enhanced by the use of a hearing aid. Nurses should encourage people who have hearing difficulties to seek appropriate aid and/or direct them to an appropriate agency. Millions of poeple already use hearing aids successfully, many more would benefit from using one.

Section II

The eye

The eye is far less complicated than we all fear. It is just an arrangement of common body tissues, some of which happen to be transparent. Together they form an organ that has only a few responses to the many insults that might come its way.

Generations of traditional teaching have described these insults at length in a strange language that turns the subject into a one-sided conflict between memory and reason. It has also turned it into a fading recollection of curious syndromes that do not always square with the hesitant signs we think we might have found.

The secret for doctor and nurse alike is to recognise the few responses—they are really quite simple—and the many causes to which they have responded will fall into the natural patterns of common pathology. These can then be worked out at leisure, because they are understood and not just remembered.

It is possible to make a fair judgment of what might be seen within the eye from what is seen without, and this is of matchless importance to the nurse faced with first post-operative dressings, with surgeons on one end of the telephone and not wanting to come to the other end, and with all those lonely decisions in the Accident and Emergency Department.

Four
The eye

Applied anatomy and physiology

Introduction

The sole purpose of the eye is to see and it does this by allowing
light to travel through a series of transparent structures to a sensitive film—the retina—which forms the inner lining of more than
half the globe. Its position, shape and behaviour are all subordinate
to this end.

It might seem that extraordinary tissues are needed to produce
this marvel, but in fact they are to be found anywhere in the body
(Fig. 4.1). Even those that are transparent resemble those that are
not more than they differ from them. The attacks of disease make

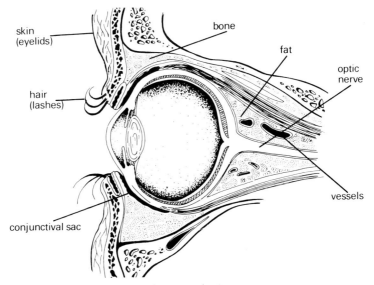

Fig. 4.1 An assembly of commonplace tissues.

this resemblance almost total, because special tissues are always prepared to cease to be special rather than to cease to be altogether.

Each eye faces forwards from a bony cavity in the skull—the orbit. Hair known as eyelashes sprouts from the margins of the eyelids, which themselves are formed of skin, fibrous plates and muscles (Fig. 4.2). A wet membrane—the conjunctiva—lines the deep surface of the lids, folding backwards on to the eye as a sac, which then unfolds forwards again to blend with that clear window at the front of the eye—the cornea.

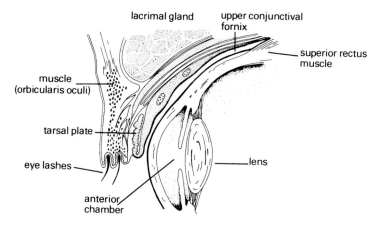

Fig. 4.2 The tear moist alliance between the eyelids, the conjunctiva and the cornea.

This membrane, threatened by dryness by the atmosphere, has to be kept moist by a salty solution which flows continually from the tear gland. A similar gland moistens the mouth. Superfluous tears drain away through little holes in the eyelids and along minute drainage channels to collect in the tear sac, whence they flow along yet another canal into the nose.

The outer coat of the eye—the sclera—is rather like the ball of a joint which moves in a socket of muscle, bone and eyelids (Fig. 4.3). It is formed of collagen fibres and suffers the same diseases as does collagen anywhere in the body.

The middle coat of the eye is a blend of blood vessels, pigment cells and muscle, woven together by connective tissue. It is visible in front as the iris, where its dappled shading has given rise to much languid poetry and not a few imprudent decisions. The hole around which the iris is arranged—the pupil—regulates the amount of

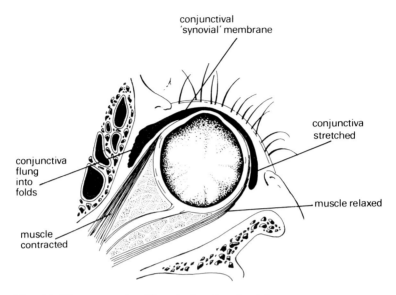

conjunctival
'synovial' membrane

conjunctiva
stretched

conjunctiva
flung
into
folds

muscle relaxed

muscle
contracted

Fig. 4.3 The eye moving like a ball and socket joint.

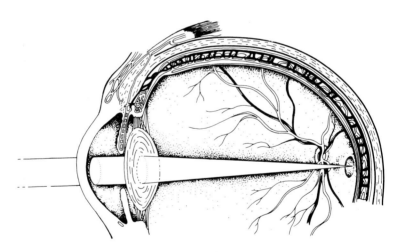

Fig. 4.4 A cone of light brought to a point of focus at the macula by the cornea and the lens.

light entering the eye, rather like the aperture of a camera (Fig. 4.4).

The iris merges backwards into the ciliary body, from which the lens dangles, and which produces the aqueous fluid that normally

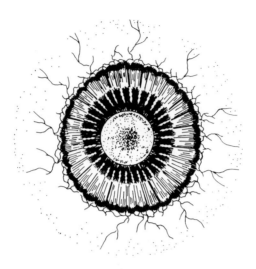

Fig. 4.5 The iris and pupil seen through the cornea and the fine
network of vessels encircling the corneo-scleral limbus and seen better if
seen closer with a small convex lens (+ lens).

circulates through the eye to maintain both its health and its shape
(Fig. 4.5).

The ciliary body itself merges backwards into the choroid, which
feeds the deep surface of the retina and is the basis of that familiar
red glow seen in the eyes of those startled by a flashlight
photographer.

The innermost coat—the retina—is part of the brain. Its refine-
ment of behaviour, whilst allowing great subtlety of perception of
light, has made reproduction of fresh retina an impossibility. It
consists in fact of two distinct layers which merge at the anterior
limit of the functioning retina, along that scalloped border between
the ciliary body and the choroid (Fig. 4.6), the ora serrata.

Of the two transparent structures within the globe the first is the
lens, which alters its shape in response to the demands of the
focusing muscles.

Behind the lens the major cavity of the globe is filled with the
second transparent substance—the vitreous body.

So much for the inside of the eye, the tissues outside, like tissues
anywhere else, deal with movement and pain sensation.

Each eye is moved by six muscles, and as there are two eyes, each
gazes on the world from a different viewpoint. The brain fuses these
separate one-dimensional views into one single view, and this two-
eyed perception in depth is called binocular vision (Fig. 4.7).

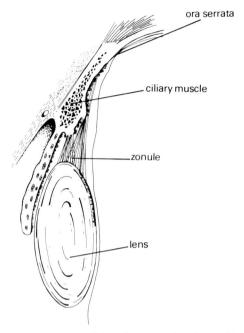

Fig. 4.6 The anterior relations of the vitreous gel and its adherence to the retina at the ora serrata.

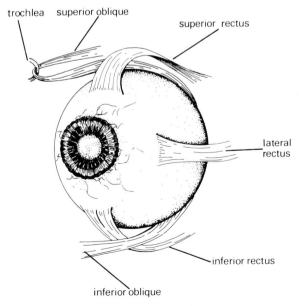

Fig. 4.7 The extra-ocular muscles of the left eye.

The rest of the orbit is filled with arteries, veins, cranial nerves and fat.

It must now be evident that the eye is just another collection of familiar tissues, unique perhaps in its shape, needlessly worrying in its entirety, but totally commonplace when each section is taken separately.

The transparent tissues

The cornea

This convex window transmits and focuses light. Like any quality refracting surface it must be smooth. To keep it this way the eyelids must blink snugly across its surface, coating it with tears and removing any unwanted debris. Anything that disrupts this arrangement puts its patrician clarity in danger of replacement by common epithelium, which is certainly tough but also opaque.

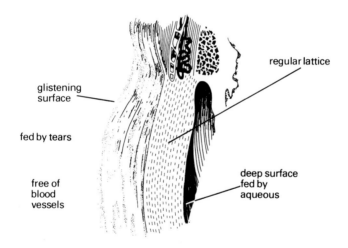

regular lattice

glistening surface

fed by tears

free of blood vessels

deep surface fed by aqueous

Fig. 4.8 How the cornea stays clear.

With a blood supply confined to its margin, the cornea derives much of its food and oxygen from tears, which do for the anterior surface of the cornea what the blood does for other tissues (Fig. 4.8). A cornea starved of atmospheric oxygen by ill-chosen contact lenses will rapidly settle for a blood-borne oxygen supply which infiltrates beyond its margin. If the starvation continues, the infiltration will continue and the clarity will not (Fig. 4.9).

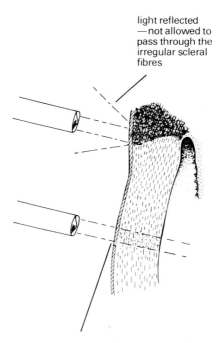

light reflected
—not allowed to
pass through the
irregular scleral
fibres

Fig. 4.9 Light is transmitted only through a regular corneal lattice.

Clarity in the deep structures of the cornea depends on their regular arrangement, and also on a reduced water content achieved by the deepest layer of all, which operates a pump to keep the cornea in a state of semihydration. Naturally, any disturbance of the deep layer—for example a deposit of inflammatory debris—will result in corneal oedema (Fig. 4.10).

The lens

Layered like an onion, but shaped like a lentil, and suspended from the ciliary body, the lens changes its convexity and hence its focusing power in response to the demands made on it by the ciliary muscles (Fig. 4.6).

Like the cornea, the lens could not remain clear and also could not remain transparent without a transparent circulation. It therefore depends on the aqueous fluid which circulates from the ciliary body as a blood substitute. Any disturbance of this aqueous fluid can jeopardise the metabolism of the lens. Any disruption of this metabolism may produce an opacity, and we call such an opacity a cataract, whatever its cause.

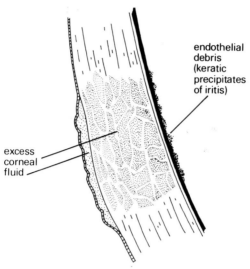

endothelial
debris
(keratic
precipitates
of iritis)

excess
corneal
fluid

Fig. 4.10 Corneal oedema. Iritic debris interfering with the suction mechanism of the endothelium.

The lens marks the division between the anterior and posterior segments of the eye.

The vitreous body

An inert whorl of collagen fibres and hyaluronic acid, the vitreous fills the cavity of the eye behind the lens. Its metabolism is languid and opacities arising from disease clear away with equal languer, if they do so at all.

The aqueous humour

All living tissue requires a circulation to stay alive. If it is opaque, then an opaque circulation like blood serves very well. But if it is transparent then the circulation must be transparent also.

The blood substitute in the eye for the transparent tissues is the aqueous fluid (Fig. 4.11). Its behaviour is so simple that most people, if they know about it at all, cannot believe that there is not something else to it. Because it has nothing so obvious as a radial pulse, it flows in secret when things are well and sadly when things are not well, and any malaise in the aqueous circulation will only come to light if we are not distracted by the claims of more florid clinical features.

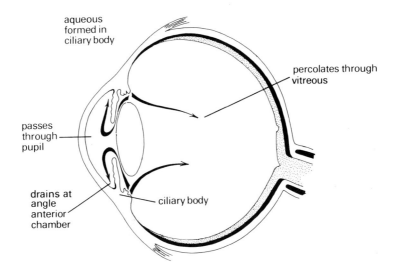

aqueous
formed in
ciliary body

percolates through
vitreous

passes
through
pupil

drains at
angle
anterior
chamber

ciliary body

Fig. 4.11 The aqueous circulation. Unsuspected when circulating well; unsuspected when not circulating well.

The aqueous is secreted by the ciliary body and flows through the pupil to fill the anterior chamber. Having done its duty as a blood substitute for the lens and the cornea it then filters out of the eye through a meshwork that lies in the angle at the anterior chamber between the iris and the cornea.

The normal eye can be thought of as a soft-walled sphere full of a liquid that forms inside and flows outside at an equal rate. This simple circulation of aqueous lies at the very core of the eye's existence. If secretion ceases, the eye will collapse. Disturbance of its contents can disturb the clear tissues of the globe dependent on it. Blockage of its circulation at any point, from its source in the ciliary body to its exit at the drainage angle, will raise the pressure of the eyeball. This raised pressure is called glaucoma and the type will vary with the cause of the blockage.

When the pressure of the eyeball rises above the pressure of the blood feeding the opaque parts of the globe, they will die eventually of ischaemia.

How the eye sees

There are two distinct kinds of normal vision—central vision and field of vision.

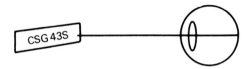

Fig. 4.12 Central vision—in the distance.

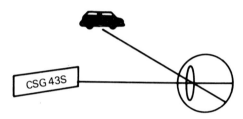

Fig. 4.13 Central vision and field of vision—in the distance.

Central vision

The ability to recognise colour and to make precise distinctions between almost similar details is served by a tiny layer of retina just lateral to the optic nerve head. This is called the macula and, to be absolutely accurate, the even tinier centre is called the fovea (Fig. 4.12 and Fig. 4.13).

It is the kind of vision that all people know about. When something goes wrong they are very quick to complain. However, they make the grievous blunder of thinking that it is the only kind of vision.

Field of vision

The other, and really more vital kind of vision—the field—gives us vast amounts of information about our surroundings and provides the central area with things to look at in detail. Served by receptor cells called rods, which come into their own in reduced illumination. This process is called dark adaptation. It is lost in some retinal diseases, the most famous of which and perhaps the most uncommon is retinitis pigmentosa.

The dark adapted retina, dependent on rods, cannot recognise colour. It is this feature which produces that subtle, yet heightened, perception in the moonlight—those honeyed shadows that daylight sharpens with an unpalatable edge.

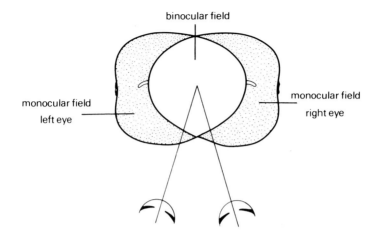

Fig. 4.14 What the eyes can see together and what they see separately.

Each eye has a visual field shaped rather like a recumbent pear, with the bulbous end pointing to the lateral side (Fig. 4.14). With both eyes open, these fileds have a binocular overlap where each eye sees the same thing at the same time. However there is a degree of independence, for the bulbous end of the pear on the temporal side provides a crescent of vision that belongs to that eye alone. This fact can be demonstrated by maintaining fixation with the central vision on some immobile distant object, whilst covering each eye alternately.

With an intact pathway running from the macula to the occipital cortex, it would be reasonable to assume that normal central vision would exist automatically. Unfortunately, as far as central vision is concerned, health alone is not enough, for central vision is not a birthright.

An intact pathway will not allow normal central vision to develop if the circumstances for this development are not favourable. A popular name for this failure is a lazy eye and one of the causes might be a childhood squint.

Because both eyes supply one binocular field, one of them may fail without there being any subjective awareness of loss from this field. As long as the central vision remains intact, people assume their eyes are healthy, whilst a disease like chronic glaucoma may be quietly nibbling away at the edges. It is the field that succumbs to a rise in pressure, while the centre survives until the very end.

Focusing mechanisms

Light does not enter the eye in a casual manner. It has to come to a focus at the macula.

Normal sight

In the relaxed state, an eye with this quality will bring rays of light from the distance (anything further than 6 metres) to a point of focus on the macula (Fig. 4.15). Normal distance visual acuity is recorded as 6/6 (20/20 feet). The upper figure is the distance at which the test card is seen. The lower figure is the distance at which the letter size ought to be seen. 6/12 means that 6 metres distance the eye in question could only make out a letter size which should have been seen at 12 metres (Fig. 4.16).

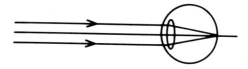

Fig. 4.15 The normal sighted eye (emmetropic). Sees in the distance without effort.

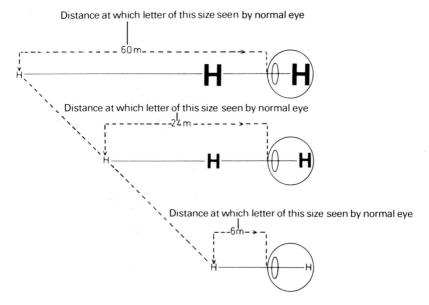

Fig. 4.16 What the fractions recorded from a Snellen chart mean.

Near vision

Similar to a camera, an eye can pull its focus from infinity to nearer than 6 metres. It achieves this by contraction of the ciliary muscle, which allows the lens to become more convex, hence shortening its focal length. The distance chosen will vary with habit, and indeed the length of the arm (Fig. 4.17). As the years go by the lens hardens, failing to respond to instructions from the ciliary muscle. Beginning in the mid-20s, this process becomes recognisable only in the mid-40s when people resist the discovery that their arms are becoming too short for visual comfort. Presbyopia is the name given to this unfortunate discovery. It increases with age, when lenses of increasing strength are required to compensate for the lost focusing power (Fig. 4.18).

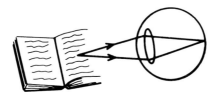

Fig. 4.17 The normal sighted eye. Focuses for near by making its lens more convex. The pupil constricts incidently at the same time.

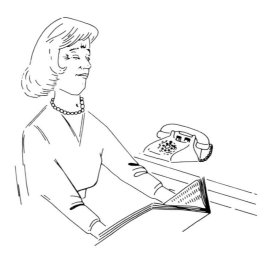

Fig. 4.18 Presbyopia—the denied evidence of advancing years.

Long sight

Long sight, or hypermetropia, is commonly thought to mean miracles of distance vision, but in fact a long-sighted eye is a small eye—indeed too small for its own relaxed focus. So, although it may see into the distance, it has to use up its reading focus to do so, and by the time it comes to focus for near, it may have used up the focus altogether (Fig. 4.19).

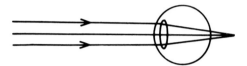

Fig. 4.19 The long sighted eye (hypermetropic). Has to make its lens more convex to see in the distance. There may be no range of focus left when it tries to see for near.

Short sight

Parallel rays of light from the distance come to focus between the lens and the retina, giving these myopic eyes a blurred hint of things of interest, but not much more. The object has to be brought closer to the eyeball so that the rays of light diverging from it will push the focusing point nearer the retina to be of use. Such eyes see near objects without effort, but they pay the price of seeing little in the distance, no matter what the effort (Fig. 4.20).

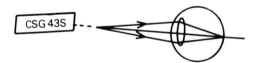

Fig. 4.20 The short sighted eye (myopic). Cannot see in the distance at all, the relaxed focus may be already close enough to the eye for effortless reading.

Astigmatism

The eye does not always focus as a perfect sphere. Such an eye can never bring rays of light to a point. They bring them to a horizontal oval and are sharp in one meridian or the other, but never in both together.

Five
Clinical features of eye disorders

What the patient complains of

As the responses of the eye to disease are few, so are the symptoms produced by these diseases. There are essentially five symptoms which the patient complains of:
1. alteration in appearance
2. pain
3. disturbance of tears
4. disturbance of vision
5. double vision.

Only the last two are strictly ophthalmic. Normal appearances can be judged by looking at the first available face. Pain can occur anywhere. The tear apparatus is just a lubricating and drainage system that happens to lie beside the eye.

Alterations in appearance

This is simply any deviation that lies outwith the wide range of what we accept as normal.

Pain

If the pain originates in the eye then it will either occur immediately the eye is used or it will be obvious beyond doubt if one takes time to listen to the patient's story.

Disturbance of the tear apparatus

Reduced tear secretion from a gland faltering with age or because of one of the rheumatic disorders cannot moisten the eye sufficiently to keep it comfortable or safe from infection.

Watering follows disruption of the flow of tears either from an ill-fitting eyelid or a blocked nasolacrimal duct. Irritation of the eyes also produces watering, even in the presence of a normal drain.

Disturbance of vision

As the eye is part of the central nervous system, visual symptoms fall into two groups:
(i) the absence of features that ought to be present,
(ii) the presence of features which ought not to be present.

Visual loss

Central vision. If patients complain of loss of vision, they usually mean loss of central vision. A cataract may stop light passing through the lens. A degenerate macula stops the light from being picked up by the central retina, even if it has managed to pass through the lens.

Field of vision. Any lesion like a tumour or an aneurysm may press upon the visual pathway. The patient is very often unaware that anything has gone wrong unless the defect is of sudden onset. The most common cause of field loss is chronic glaucoma, which quietly erodes the visual field of one eye, whilst normal central vision of both and an intact field of one lull patients into a false sense of security.

Occasional transient loss of vision may follow variations in the central blood flow. When someone rises from a crouching position, with the head moving faster than the blood, then one of the first symptoms is a dimness of vision. A similar loss is noticed as a prelude to a faint, and, of course, pathologically when the blood supply to the head is insufficient for the demands of normal activity.

Abnormal visual sensations

Haloes. If the cornea's dehydrating mechanism falters, the patient will be aware of the colours of the rainbow shaped in a ring around lights. This is a classic warning of an imminent attack of acute glaucoma (Ch. 10). Haloes of one colour alone occur when some opacity, usually a cataract, interferes with the passage of light.

Flashing lights. The visual pathway from the retina to the brain is a system designed to produce some precise form of light sensation in response to visual impulses. It produces less precise forms of light sensation to other impulses, which may range from breaks in the retina to tumours in the temporal lobe of the brain.

Floaters. Normal degenerations of the vitreous jelly, happening in the fullness of time, leave little strands and wisps in the vitreal cavity that become visible, and often a trial, to their possessor. Other floaters develop in response to disease. They all tend to appear the same to the patient, but the sudden onset of new floaters would tend to suggest that something has happened recently. What has happened may be a break in the retina or some process of scattering opaque debris, like blood or inflammatory material, through the eye.

Double vision. Allegations of double vision frequently turn out to be simple blurring. However, genuine double vision can mean one of two things.
1. If it occurs with only one eye open then something, usually a cataract, has split the light entering the eye-monocular diplopia.
2. If it happens with both eyes open then some opacity may still have split the light in one eye, but more likely the eyes will have suddenly begun to point in different directions. The commonest cause for this is a paralysed muscle.

Patients who have squinted since childhood cannot experience real double vision because their eyes have never learned to work at the same time. They look with one eye but suppress the vision of the other.

How to elicit essential signs

Ophthalmic examination can be reduced to a handful of simple elements. It can be agreed that a careful look at a normal face may give a standard base line against which any variations can be measured. Thereafter we require a way of determining whether failure to see will respond to a pair of glasses or not. This is perfectly possible without a box of lenses and a grasp of optics. It may be the first step to a diagnosis, for it is mandatory to explain why a patient does not see as well as he ought to, or used to.

We then need to know the state of the visual field.

We require signs that will allow us to distinguish the serious causes of a red eye from the less serious causes, and all of them from each other—without ambiguity.

The pressure of the eyeball can be estimated roughly without instruments.

Finally we come to the ophthalmoscope, which allows a view of the posterior pole of the eyeball. On practical grounds this means the optic disc, the macula and the adjacent blood vessels. All too often we gaze into the eye hoping for a diagnosis to emerge, and in fact all that we find is a further reason to doubt the diagnosis that we already think we have made.

The secret of ophthalmic examination is to establish from the examination outside what you expect to find inside.

The pin-hole disc

This ridiculously cheap instrument works on a very simple principle. As the rays of light presented to an eye, all bar the central one, are deviated out of line by the focusing bar of that eye (Fig. 5.1A and Fig. 5.1B). The central ray, however, is never deviated, because there is nothing to deviate it, and so it must reach the macula, no matter what the refractive error is. In normal circumstances the fact of its passage is overwhelmed by all the other rays that move people to say they cannot see. However, the pin-hole disc eliminates them all, leaving the central ray to pass on its own.

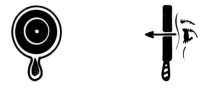

Fig. 5.1A The pinhole disc (An infallible method to tell if poor central vision (for distance and near) is due to a spectacle error or not.).

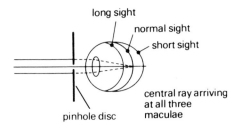

Fig. 5.1B How the pinhole disc works.

If the macula has the potential to see it, then the pin-hole disc will prove it. This can be done for distance with a Snellan chart, or for near with any scrap of print that comes to hand. The visual pathways run anatomically from the retinae along the optic nerves, the optic chiasma, the optic tracts and the optic radiation, to the occipital cortex of the brain. Each visual field is split into a temporal half and a nasal half, the divide taking place vertically through the fixing point of central vision—the macula. The temporal half of each retina is represented by the visual cortex of its own side. The nasal part of each retina passes over to the opposite side at the optic chiasma. The relationship of this chiasma to the pituitary gland and the large intra-cranial blood vessels may be reflected in visual field loss when these structures become bigger than they ought to.

In general terms, lesions anterior to the chiasma must affect one eye. Lesions at the chiasma damage the crossing fibres, whilst lesions behind the chiasma catch temporal fibres from one side plus the nasal fibres from the opposite side.

Confrontation field

Only the hands are required to perform this test. The patient is asked to cover one eye and to look directly at the eye of the examiner. All we then need to do is to trace out the pear-shaped field with both hands together. This is a rough screening test, but certainly not so rough as to be useless. Should it reveal any defect, then of course this defect must be examined formally.

Such formal examination involves presenting targets of different colour and size against a standard background in a standard illumination. Each eye is tested separately and of course as nearly immobile as natural curiosity might allow (Fig. 5.2).

With good co-operation it is possible to chart the exact dimensions of the normal field for a given target size and a given illumination. And with the same variables in mind it is equally possible to give an exact description of the abnormal field, particularly those areas of less than perfect vision.

The eye itself

From the long catalogue of signs declared by tradition to be vital, there are in fact only two observations to be made and a third subtle one. As the first leads on to the second and the third lies between the two, they can be held easily by the shortest of memories:
1. The state of the cornea

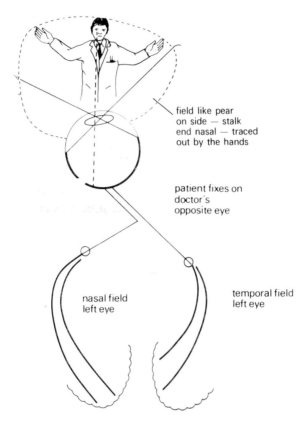

field like pear
on side — stalk
end nasal — traced
out by the hands

patient fixes on
doctor's
opposite eye

nasal field
left eye

temporal field
left eye

Fig. 5.2 How to test the visual field by confrontation. As important as
the pinhole disc. If the doctor tries to cover one of his own eyes he will
find himself attempting with two hands a manoeuvre for which he
clearly needs three. The ensuing charade may be too much for the
patients.

2. The state of the pupil
3. The depth of the anterior chamber.

Corneal lustre

The cornea glistens and sparkles in youth, although turning with
ill-health and age into the familiar lacklustre eyes of the elderly, as
though decades of watching human activity had dulled the eyes as
well as the spirits. Breaches in the anterior surface of the cornea
may be picked up with a dye—sodium fluorescein. Such breaches,
of course, open a channel for infection to the cavity of the eye and

raise the risk of disturbing the regular corneal lattice arrangement with permanent effects on vision.

The state of the pupil

The pupil has two muscles. The more powerful, a sphincter running round its margin, makes the pupil smaller in response to light and it relaxes in order to allow the pupil to become bigger when illumination is reduced.

Active constriction passes via the parasympathetic nervous system.

The weaker muscle, the dilater, radiates to the periphery of the iris from the pupil margin and is mediated through the sympathetic nervous system. It explains the dilatation of the pupils from anxiety and terror (Fig. 5.3).

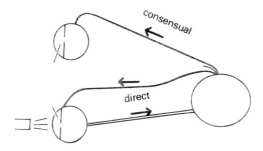

Fig. 5.3 The pupil light reaction. Both respond when one is exposed to a bright light.

The depth of the anterior chamber

Eclipse test. The anterior chamber is that area lying between the iris and the cornea. A shallow anterior chamber may interfere with the free flow of aqueous through the drain in the angle of the anterior chamber. An eye with such a shallow chamber is liable to acute glaucoma (Fig. 5.4).

To detect it, a light is directed from the margin of the cornea across the place of the iris. In a safe, deep chamber the entire iris will be suffused with light. In the dangerous shallow kind, only the half adjacent to the light will be illuminated. The remote half will be in shadow. The light is eclipsed. The pupil of such an eye must not be dilated.

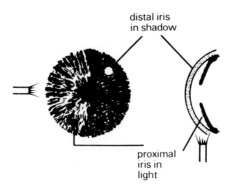

distal iris
in shadow

proximal
iris in
light

Fig. 5.4 The eclipse test. Failure to observe whether or not the anterior chamber is shallow is negligence.

Intra-ocular pressure. Thoughts of acute glaucoma should put us in mind of a tense eyeball with more aqueous than it can cope with. It should also remind us that a raised pressure has to be considered every time we look at an eye and that most raised pressures are not caused by acute glaucoma.

Digital tonometry. (Fig. 5.5). The basic principle is to palpate the eyeball for fluctuation, rather like a boil. However, it is more useful to palpate the eye and not the tarsal plate. Palpation must therefore be done above the tarsal plate, with the eye looking downwards. This allows us to touch the eyeball through the thinnest part of the eyelid. The pressure is then estimated with the fingers. The easiest way is to lean on the patient's forehead with the ring fingers, brushing the pulp of the one index finger against the nail of the other, whilst both fingers are in contact with the globe. Clearly this is not indicated on an eye which has just undergone surgery.

Looking at the fundus. Ophthalmology began effectively in the middle of the 19th century when Helmholtz rediscovered what the medical press had ignored 30 years before when it was first described by Purkinje—a man whose entire life seems to have been spent making medical discoveries in Czech that have brought fame to others in French, German and English.

In principle, light is introduced through the pupil to illuminate the back of the eye. The illuminated fundus is then viewed through a small aperture, which allows the observer to be aware of the light flowing outwards from the eye. In general, little information can be achieved through a small pupil, yet there is no well-known

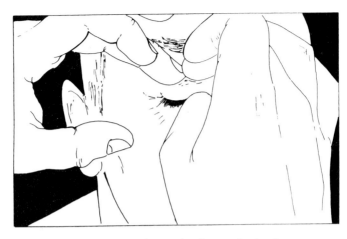

Fig. 5.5 Finger tension. Ring fingers leaning on forehead; pressure taken by middle or index fingers—palpating globe like a boil above outer margin of tarsal plate. The fingers are brushed together alternatively pulp to nail.

precise rule about when it is safe to dilate the pupil—only an imprecise vague terror about when not to. The eclipse test should eliminate all such uncertainty. It is not enough to leave these decisions to the doctor. If the nurse is to be involved at all in ophthalmic care, then such basic rules must be understood.

A safe eye

A safe eye is one that does not harbour some preventable, but as yet undetected, blinding disease. Most conditions draw attention to themselves one way or another. There are, however, two sinister conditions where a patient with intact central vision can be re-assured that all is well, only to be told a year later that all is not well. And there is a third, where a patient may return in some pain rather sooner.

The first is any situation where the pressure of the eyeball is raised, the most common being chronic glaucoma. The second, more rare, is a space-occupying lesion of the pituitary fossa. Both nibble away at that portion of the vision that people are least aware of—the field.

The third condition is a shape rather than a disease, namely the eye with a shallow anterior chamber—symptomless until it explodes into an attack of acute glaucoma.

The above system will uncover positive signs where there are those to be uncovered. Although it may not always tell what *is* wrong, it will always tell what *is not* wrong, and if an eye can be described as safe—with confidence—then the plaintive request by doctor or nurse for an urgent ophthalmic opinion might turn into a more confident statement that it can wait, if indeed it is at all necessary.

Six
Basic principles in a special organ

Introduction

The greatest obstacle to simplicity is the firm belief held by every speciality that it is unique, with a special language and a special importance that places it apart from the common run of all other specialities. Sovereign remedies, nostrums, ancient traditions and syndromes named after some bearded sage of another era, all took the place of a rationale basis of treatment, and sadly sometimes continue to do so. There is in fact a limited range of things that can actually go wrong. It is the local variations that make them seem that inexhaustible. All tissues can suffer congenital defects, tumours, inflammation, vascular disturbances and so on. Regional differences add a touch of local colour, but they do not change the basic processes.

As an example, inflammation whatever its cause or whatever its site, can give rise to redness, swelling, pain, heat and loss of function. It may then disappear. It may leave marks of damage in its wake, or may grumble on as a chronic destructive process. If this happens in the iris, then of course it is an ophthalmic problem, but it is still inflammation.

Inflammation of the iris

In this chapter, using iritis as an example, an explanation of how symptoms and signs can be worked out on a reasoned basis, and how on the same basis a logical system of management can be applied, is given (Fig. 6.1).

The clinical features and management of an inflammatory attack on the iris can be worked out from a basic knowledge of pathophysiology.
1. The blood vessels at the margin of the cornea become inflamed—the only vessels linked to the iris vessels that are visible on the outside.

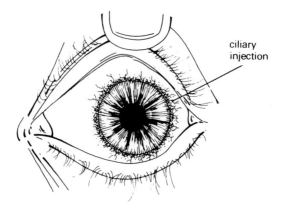

ciliary
injection

Fig. 6.1 Iritis. One of the three major red eyes showing inflammation around the corneo-scleral limbus and possibly nothing else.

2. The iris swells exuding debris into the anterior chamber. This is the equivalent of oedema.
3. The muscles of the iris sphincter go into spasm, producing a small pupil and some degree of pain.
4. Inflammatory material dancing about in the visual field can cause tantalising visual disturbance. This inflammatory material can also become deposited in the angle of the anterior chamber, so blocking the flow of aqueous fluid.
5. As the inflammation proceeds adhesions may develop between the adjacent structures, most usually the iris and the lens.
6. The toxic aqueous may disturb the lens metabolism, producing a cataract (Fig. 6.2).

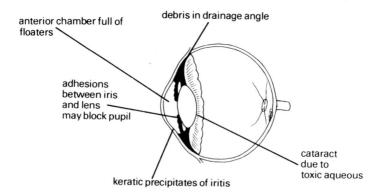

anterior chamber full of floaters

debris in drainage angle

adhesions between iris and lens may block pupil

keratic precipitates of iritis

cataract due to toxic aqueous

Fig. 6.2 Iritis. The possible complications; obstruction of the aqueous flow may not be suspected until the visual field is impaired.

Clinical findings related to pathology

These can also be understood if we just pause a minute or two and think about the pathology and the organ involved.

1. Central vision may be affected.
2. The field of vision will be normal.
3. The cornea should be clear in the early stages. If the deep surface is coated with inflammatory debris then the overlying cornea will be waterlogged, appearing to the patient and observer to be very much like the translucency of water hosing down a fishmonger's window.
4. The pupil will be small and spastic, unless distorted by a previous attack.
5. The anterior chamber depth should be normal. However, a shallow anterior chamber could well indicate that the patient suffers from acute glaucoma, with iris inflammation as a secondary condition.

Principles of medical/surgical treatment

As with clinical examination, schemes of management are the same whatever organ is involved. We can reduce the scheme to a series of principles common to all branches of medicine. These may be divided into medical or surgical—short term or long term.

1. The exciting cause should be removed if possible.
2. The destructive process should be curbed if possible.
3. The complications should be anticipated. It should be remembered that remedies frequently have complications also.
4. Restoration of function is hopefully the end product of therapeutic intervention.

Short-term treatment

Corticosteroids are the time honoured drug used to suppress inflammation of unknown origin. The frequency of dosage must be tailored to the severity of the condition. Four times a day in the treatment of ophthalmic conditions has somehow acquired an almost scriptural sanctity, but in many cases four times an hour might be more appropriate, if the drugs are to be effective in resolving the disorder. It is not out of place to mention at this point that long-term abuse of corticosteroids may be as toxic to the eye as the disease itself. They raise the intra-ocular pressure and open the door to infection.

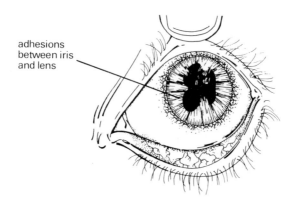

adhesions
between iris
and lens

Fig. 6.3 Iritis. Adhesion between the iris and the lens. Atropine does not stop this but it does make the adhesions work harder if they are to block the entire pupil.

Inflammation produces adhesions and if the entire pupil margin is stuck down then vision will eventually be affected, whilst the aqueous drainage will be immediately so. This complication can often be prevented by dilating the pupil. A drug commonly used is atropine 1%. The twice daily application of atropine drops may adequately achieve such dilatation (Fig. 6.3).

The effects of atropine have been known for centuries. The other name of 'belladonna' derives from the custom of Roman ladies of fashion who added lustre to their eyes by dilating their pupils. They considered that limpid pools, black beneath tremulous lashes, were seductive. This was probably true, and for the ladies had the matchless advantage of blurring away the deformities of their more misshapen consorts!

If the aqueous circulation has been blocked then the intra-ocular pressure will rise and will need to be brought down. One of the drugs most commonly used to do this is azetazolamide, another is dichlorophenamide (Ch. 15). In the short term we are not generally concerned with perfect function, but we should not forget that the patient will want to use the eye again.

There is frequently pain which varies considerably from mild discomfort to severe pain. The pain will often decrease when the mydriatic begins to effectively dilate the pupil. However, some patients will require analgesics, whilst some may even require a narcotic agent. Pain relief may also be gained by applying warm compresses or by 'hot spoon' bathing (Ch. 7).

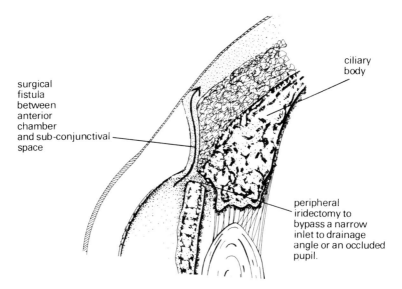

ciliary
body

surgical
fistula
between
anterior
chamber
and sub-conjunctival
space

peripheral
iridectomy to
bypass a narrow
inlet to drainage
angle or an occluded
pupil.

Fig. 6.4 The essence of a glaucoma operation.

Long-term treatment

This applies only to the complications of a smouldering chronic iritis. If the pressure of the eye remains high following the disease this will have to be kept under control with long-term anti-glaucoma therapy. If medical therapy fails then it will be necessary to attempt surgical treatment.

This involves cutting a hole in the sclera to allow aqueous to drain from the eye (Fig. 6.4). Such a manoeuvre is an outrage to the body, which naturally tries to close over the hole, and indeed it frequently succeeds, especially in an eye that already has a tendency to inflammatory scarring. If the blockage is at the pupil then a hole may also be cut in the iris to allow the aqueous to escape through the the normal drain at the anterior chamber angle. For some reason the iris never attempts to heal over these perforations.

Should the lens have succumbed either to the disease or treatment, then a cataract extraction may be indicated (Ch. 9).

Discussion

Whatever the basic pathology, the patient will respond with a limited number of symptoms, and the eye with a limited number of signs. Awareness of the normal aqueous flow will warn us to beware, because the flow may well cease to be normal with no obvious signs at all. The ritual of examination will tell us what is wrong or what is not wrong. The principles of management, not unique to the eye, will tell us how to put it right if that is possible. It might also warn us that just because someone recovers while taking some medication or other, that does not necessarily mean that he recovered because he was taking it. There is now, however, no reason why we cannot begin to predict what can go wrong with an eye, more to the point what can be done about it, and above all provide a common ground for discussions with the doctors involved.

Nursing aspects

Nurses caring for the patient with iritis must administer the prescribed medical treatment and observe the effects of the medication and the patient's condition in general.

Because of the disorder and the dilated pupils the patient will have some disturbance of vision and must be nursed accordingly. Most patients will be extremely anxious so that reassurance is essential. The doctor will indicate whether he wishes the patient to remain in bed, with bathroom privileges, or whether he may be more active. Patients should also be warned about bending over, and straining at the stool should be prevented by the judicious use of dietary fibre or a laxative. Should the patient complain of any increased pain the doctor should be informed, as this may be an indication of complications developing, such as a secondary glaucoma. Most patients should be be able to be up and about and, provided they take care, will come to no harm. Treatment has usually to continue after discharge so that either the patient or his relatives must be carefully instructed on how to instill the drops/ointment as prescribed (see Ch. 16).

Seven
The external eye

The eyelids, the conjunctiva and the cornea form a natural alliance working together in health and failing to work together in disease. The ill effects of this failure tends to spread from the more robust eyelids to the less robust conjunctiva, and finally to the least robust of all—the cornea. The cornea tends to keep its problems to itself, or it may pass them deeper still to involve the iris, whence they may spread to involve the whole interior of the globe.

The extreme sensitivity of the cornea forces all but the most phlegmatic of patients to complain at least of some discomfort. All the available symptoms can appear, but not all at once. Relevant complaints can be confirmed by simple observation. Understanding of the signs is also elementary. The secret is to look at all eyes in the same way every time.

Disorders of the external eye

Principles of treatment

The health of the outer eye relies on eyelids snugly fitting, puncta inward, lashes outward, and actively blinking—spreading tears from a moist abundant conjunctiva sac over a smooth transparent cornea. Anything that maintains or restores this arrangement without recourse to frank charlatanry can be called treatment.

Medications of one sort or another can be applied to the eye as drops or ointment. Higher concentrations can be achieved by injection underneath the conjunctiva. Systemic dosage may reinforce local treatment. Surgery comes as a last resort or when the condition is due to some distortion of the normal anatomy.

Drops. Although these have a long and celebrated history, they are not the most efficient way of applying a high concentration of the required drug. The tears rapidly dilute and wash away the drug so that effective concentrations are only maintained for a short period. This is unlikely to influence bacterial frolics which go on all day. Indeed it may even lead to the development of resistant strains of bacteria (see Ch. 15).

Ointments. The major portion is a base of petroleum jelly or liquid paraffin. The more easily soluble the agent, the more effective it will be—and for longer. If over-used, ointments tend to retard the very corneal epithelium regrowth that they seek to promote. Ointments do cause some misting of vision which may be a slight disadvantage in daytime use.

Infections

A wide range of micro-organisms can produce infective inflammation. The most common bacterial infections are the *Diplococcus pneumoniae* and *Staphylococcus aureus*. Herpes simplex is the most common viral infection.

The treatment of the infection depends on its cause. In general, antibiotics are over-used and mixtures of antibiotics and corticosteroids have no place in the treatment of eye disease. The rule is the same as that which applies to inflammation elsewhere. Bacterial infections must be treated intensively with the appropriate antibiotic. Viral infections must be treated with antiviral agents (Ch. 15).

Non-specific inflammation is frequently due to tear deficiency, and if the eye is dry the answer must be to moisten it with one of the many proprietary brands of artificial tears which all tend to be based on methylcellulose (Ch. 15). Other inflammations, possibly due to allergy or to causes remote from our understanding, can be treated with anti-allergic drops such as sodium cromoglycate. Finally, when all else has failed, corticosteroid preparations may be used, but not for too long. Corticosteroids must never be instilled into the conjunctival sac until sodium fluorescein has proved the corneal epithelium to be intact.

Symptomatic relief can be achieved in some conditions by the application of warm compresses or hot spoon bathing. Analgesics for pain relief may also be required in some conditions.

The eyelids

The eyelids are the mobile part of that protective screen which stretches from the orbital margin to the eyelashes. The outer portion is formed of a delicate elastic skin, which pays the price for its enormous mobility by developing oedema easily in ill health and maddening wrinkles as the years go by. Deep to the skin lies a circular muscle—the orbicularis oculi—which closes the eye. If the nerve supply is impaired, as in a Bell's palsy, the eye will be exposed. Sensation travels along the ophthalmic division of the trigenmial nerve. The eye has to open as well as close and the upper eyelid is raised by the levator palpebra muscle, which is related closely to the superior rectus muscle.

Malposition of the eyelids

When the eyelids fail to maintain their snug relationship with the globe, then a major link in the arrangement of normality is broken and the fragile structures dependent on this arrangement begin to suffer. Should the eyelids turn outwards (ectropion), the eye is exposed (Fig. 7.1). Should the eye turn inwards (entropion), then the abrading lashes grind over the cornea like a scouring pad.

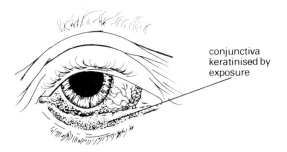

conjunctiva
keratinised by
exposure

Fig. 7.1 Ectropion. A breach in the alliance of the anterior segment. When the eyelid turns in (entropion) abrasion is substituted for exposure, but the end result is the same.

Treatment. The fragile tissues must be saved first. Infection is treated with intensive local antibiotics and corneal exposure soothed with artificial tears. Thereafter, the lids must be restored as near as possible to the flawless perfection of youth. Special attention must be given to the lid margin and to the lacrimal canaliculus, where maladroit repair can impose further elements on a problem sufficiently difficult to begin with.

Tarsal cyst

The ducts of the tarsal glands carry lubricating fluid to the deep surface of the eyelids and occasionally one of them may block. The gland contents then become stagnant and possibly infected and so present with all the well-known signs of inflammation (Fig. 7.2).

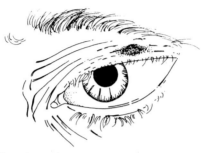

Fig. 7.2 An infected tarsal cyst. A meibomian abscess frequently mistaken for a stye.

Treatment. During the acute phase the treatment is directed towards resolving the inflammation. Intensive local antibiotics and heat in the form of hot spoon bathing (p. 134) is generally effective in relieving the inflammation. Once the infection has settled, by treatment or spontaneously, it may still leave a lump on the eyelid which will require to be incised and the contents curetted.

Rodent ulcer

This basal cell carcinoma is the most common tumour of the eyelids (Fig. 7.3). It is recognised as a dimpled lump with rolled edges and

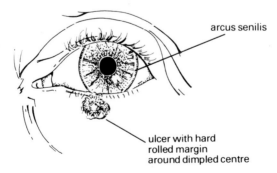

arcus senilis

ulcer with hard
rolled margin
around dimpled centre

Fig. 7.3 A rodent ulcer (basal cell carcinoma). The white arcus senilis is an unrelated reminder that the likely victim is beyond middle age.

an indolent or recurring infection that never seems to get better. If left to its own devices it can penetrate deep into the skull bones destroying everything in its wake. It is sensitive to radiotherapy and can also be treated by simple excision.

Epicanthus

A vertical fold of skin hiding the medial end of the eyelids can give the false impression of a convergent squint (Ch. 11).

Ptosis

In this disorder the upper lid fails to rise above the pupil line so that the lid appears to droop. The explanation varies with age, the mode of onset and any associated features. It may be congenital or acquired (Fig. 7.4).

The congenital variety is clearly more likely in children, although adults may have to put up with it for a long time. If the lid obscures the visual line it may threaten the development of binocular vision. Structures that defy gravity in youth tend to droop with age, and the upper lid is a classic example. Both congenital and senile ptosis are usually characterised by the total absence of sinister symptoms and by any affection of the central nervous system.

The sudden onset of a dropped lid means that something has gone wrong, either with the third cranial nerve or with the cervical sympathetic chain, frequently at the root of the neck. A third nerve palsy makes the eye virtually immobile and the pupil widely

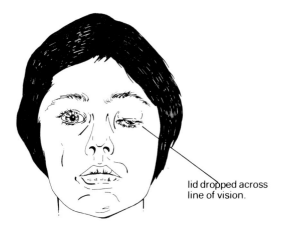

lid dropped across line of vision.

Fig. 7.4 Ptosis.

dilated, and raises the disturbing possibility of an intracranial aneurysm. The treatment of an acquired ptosis depends on its cause. Relief of pressure on the third cranial nerve may lead to complete recovery.

The eyelashes

Stye. Infection of one lash root forms the classical stye (Fig. 7.5). Chronic infection of more than one lash root is called blepharitis. Treatment is local antibiotics, and hot spoon bathing may be soothing. Before instilling the antibiotics, the scales shed by blepharitis must be removed once or twice daily (see Ch. 16) to allow the antibiotic to penetrate. Patients with recurrent styes should have their urine tested for sugar in case they have developed diabetes mellitus.

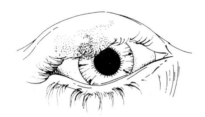

Fig. 7.5 Stye. Infection of a lash root.

The conjunctiva

The conjunctiva is that translucent lining which acts as the 'synovial membrane' for the part of the eyeball which has to make its movements exposed to air. The most common conjunctival response to insult is inflammation, and the commonest insult is bacterial infection. Drying out of the tear secretion makes the conjunctiva inflamed in its own right and can produce a fertile breeding ground for invading micro-organisms. When a normally wet membrane dries out it produces a feeling of grittiness and not surprisingly dryness—rather like the sensation in the throat after a night spent with an open mouth.

Treatment depends on the cause and includes antibiotics, artificial tears and where the conjunctiva is exposed, surgery. Some patients may require to wear protective glasses; e.g. where the nerve supply is deficient.

Subconjunctival haemorrhage

This condition often occurs spontaneously and is recognised by the total obliteration of vascular markings. No treatment is required. The patient should be reassured that the condition will clear away over a few days. If it is recurrent and bilateral, and associated with haemorrhages elsewhere, then the patient should be referred to a physician for further investigations.

Spring catarrh

This allergic condition begins in early life and tends to improve during the mid-teens (Fig. 7.6). More common perhaps in those children unfortunate enough to suffer from eczema and/or asthma, it produces giant papillae on the deep surface of the eyelids that threaten the corneal surface and occasionally abrade it into an ulcer. This is one of the few conditions where corticosteroids may be used in the presence of a broken epithelium.

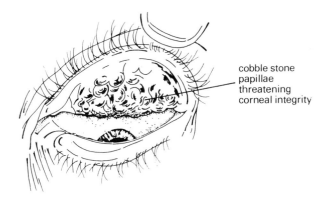

cobble stone
papillae
threatening
corneal integrity

Fig. 7.6 Spring catarrh. Part of the infantile eczema-asthma syndrome. One of the exceptional conditions where hydrocortisone may be applied in the presence of a staining cornea.

Concretions

This is really eyelid gravel—formed by persistent epithelium which ought to have been shed by the tarsal conjunctiva. It hardens into little white deposits on the deep surface of the lids. The patient complains of grittiness in the eyes. The concretions can be scraped away with a needle after a drop of local anaesthetic.

Disorders of the cornea

Any breach of the corneal epithelium may be fairly called keratitis, whether it be due to a superficial foreign body, an abrasion or an infection. It is also vital to make certain from the history whether or not something was travelling fast enough to penetrate the globe.

Herpes simplex

This infection by the herpes simplex virus can produce permanent loss of corneal clarity. Spreading from local reservoirs of infection, either a cold sore, the upper respiratory tract or indeed the conjunctiva itself, the virus settles in the corneal epithelium causing a classically branching appearance (Fig. 7.7). It may be treated with an antiviral agent such as Acyclovir (Ch. 16). It may not be treated with corticosteroids.

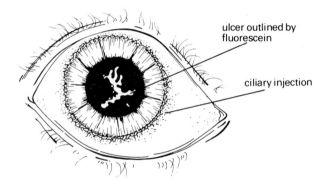

ulcer outlined by fluorescein

ciliary injection

Fig. 7.7 Dendritic ulcer. The condition where NO form of cortisone may be applied in the presence of a staining cornea.

Superficial corneal foreign bodies

Casual fragments on the corneal surface may be removed, under local drop anaesthesia, using either a moistened cotton-tipped applicator or a broad gauged needle. The casualty needs to be warned that his eye will remain insensitive for some time. A protective pad is advisable until sensation returns.

Corneal erosion

Recurrent erosion of the corneal epithelium frequently follows injury—not least an unexpected little hand across a mother's admiring eyes. The epithelium dislodged from its deep connection adheres instead overnight to the eyelid, which then rips it off in the morning. The pain is fearful, and when the patient has recovered after a few days the whole cycle may begin again.

Pinpoint erosions of the cornea develop after exposure to ultraviolet light, either radiating from a welder's torch or bouncing off the snow, to produce the well-known snow blindness. A more moderate version of the same condition is acquired by the impatient individual who attempts to acquire a 'summer tan' in a winter solarium. The same erosions may also develop as a result of broken or absent epithelium.

These lesions cannot be made to heal. They will only heal if the circumstances are favourable, and in their own time. Closure of the eyelid in the first instance with micropore tape is the best way to create these favourable circumstances. If this fails then closure of the lids with sutures may be required (tarsorrhaphy).

Conditions that cross the boundaries between the lids, the conjunctiva and the cornea

Shingles

Infection with the chicken-pox virus (varicella) causes vesiculation along any branch of the trigeminal nerve, and hence it crosses the boundaries between the lids, the conjunctiva, the cornea and the iris (Fig. 7.8). These vesicles change to pustules and form thick tenacious crusts, which appear in crops and sprays over the forehead and upper lids. They may affect the conjunctiva and the cornea, and the inflammation may spread deeper still into the iris. This does not have to affect all three every time.

It is perfectly simple now to work out what might happen. The conjunctivitis is a viral conjunctivitis which clearly does not respond to local antibiotics, although as with many virus infections, a secondary infection with bacteria may flourish.

When the cornea is affected, the position of the ulcer will determine what effect it has on vision. It tends to be sufficiently widespread to affect the vision every time. This is another occasion when local corticosteroids, contrary to ophthalmic wisdom, are indicated in the presence of a broken corneal epithelium.

The iritis of shingles, of course, is the same as iritis anywhere else, but one complicated by keratitis. In the acute phase it may produce adhesions between the iris and the lens; it may silt up the drainage angle, producing a sudden rise of intra-ocular pressure secondary to shingles iritis.

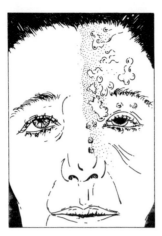

Fig. 7.8 Herpes zoster ophthalmicus. Dermatitis of the upper eyelid, conjunctivitis, keratitis, iritis—four red eyes all caused by the same thing and all self-evident. Glaucoma secondary to the iritis is also common but not self-evident.

In the long term the same debris and inflammatory damage to the meshwork of the draining angle may produce a chronic rise of intra-ocular pressure which, like all chronic rises of pressure, is discovered only if it is suspected. In addition, adhesions between the iris and the lens may produce the same effect, but at a different point in the aqueous circulation.

The poisoned aqueous can disturb lens metabolism and produce a cataract.

The skin condition may take several months to heal, leaving thin shiny epidermis where once there were pustules.

Shingles elsewhere has been called 'the girdle of roses from hell'. As far as the eye is concerned, the word 'girdle' might not be appropriate, but its source without doubt is. The pain may grumble on for months, driving its unfortunate sufferer to the point of suicide. Early treatment with systemic acyclovir may thwart the whole sequence.

Trachoma

The commonest cause of blindness in the Third World is due to this infection caused by a micro-organism (*Chlamydia trachomatis*) which lies half way between bacteria and viruses. It produces blindness by obliterating the tear inflow ducts in the upper conjunctival fornix, by scarring the cornea and by so distorting the lids that the whole alliance of the anterior segment is broken. It is a disease of filth and squalor so that amelioration of the environment is the first essential in eradicating the disease. However, we live in a less than perfect world and all too often we are left to deal with the ravages of disorder. Treatment in the acute phase with tetracyclines in an oil-based suspension is most effective. This is continued over several months. Once the disease has produced its ill effects then they can be removed in order. If the eye is dry then it can be moistened with artificial tears (Ch. 16). If the lids are turned in the wrong direction, they can be turned surgically in the right direction. If the cornea is scarred then the scar can be removed and the defect restored by a corneal graft. All of this is possible but all of this is not always available.

Third World diseases are not all due to infection. Nutritional inadequacies of all kinds produce their own types of malfunction. The classic deficiency of vitamin A leads to destruction of the corneal epithelium, whilst deficiency in the B group adversely affects nerve conduction.

Pterygium

This is a degenerative accumulation of tissues in the deep layers of the conjunctiva found along the line of the opening eyelids. More common perhaps in Europeans living in tropical exile, the condition is benign until it threatens to move across the cornea. Adopting the form of a wing, hence its name, it may relentlessly advance over the cornea from one side to the other, trailing a scar across the pupil line (Fig. 7.9).

It is evident from portraits of Admiral Nelson of Trafalgar fame, and from recorded observations of his friends that this was the cause of his poor vision and not the French guns. The only cure is surgery. This is necessary only when the wing crosses the corneal frontier.

Rosacea

This metabolic disturbance which produces blotchy inflammation over the cheeks and nose may also effect the eyes, producing the same blotchy inflammation in the conjunctiva and tongue-shaped inflammatory changes across the cornea itself. Local treatment can be worked out from what has been said before, and clearly should be started before cornea scars have diminished the vision and made local drop therapy useless.

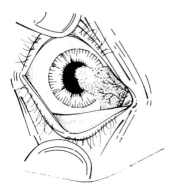

Fig. 7.9 Pterygium. A wing-like growth which threatens corneal clarity. It should be excised when it is still threatening and not when it has reached this stage.

The systemic aspects in recent years have apparently responded to long-term low usages of tetracycline. A total ban on alcohol, hot foods and other pleasing diversions has also been recommended, although there is no record that colonial administrators sustained on a diet of burra pegs and fierce curries had a higher reputation for blotchy faces than did their more abstemious counterparts at home.

Disorders of the lacrimal system

The eyes could not survive without tears, yet when the lacrimal system is upset it is the watering that people complain about most bitterly.

There are two basic kinds of tear flow: firstly, the basal production which is necessary to keep the conjunctival 'synovial' membrane healthy, and secondly a reflex flood in response to some disturbance—like a foreign body or finger in the eye. If the basal flow be diminished the ensuring grittiness may stimulate the remaining glandular cells into activity and the eye occasionally responds to tear deficiency paradoxically by watering. The drainage system from the eyelids to the nose depends not only on patency but on snug contact between the eyelid and the eyeball (Fig. 7.9).

Blockage of tear ducts

Imperforate duct. In children, a membrane at the lower end of the nasolacrimal duct occasionally remains imperforate. It is possible

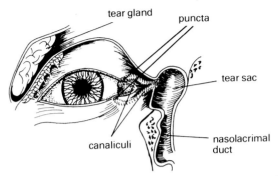

Fig. 7.10 The lacrimal appratus. A dry eye is more common than a watering one. Poorly positioned puncta are a common cause of a watering eye than is a blocked nasolacrimal duct.

to clear this membrane by probing the duct under general anaesthesia.

Chronic nasal catarrh. Blockage in adults is a not uncommon occurrence in our temperate climate, and as often as not related to chronic nasal catarrh. The great reservoir for tears is the lacrimal sac which may explode into a lacrimal abscess, classically recognised as an angry red swelling between the nose and the eyelids.

Treatment and nursing care

As specimen of the nasal discharge should be collected for culture and sensitivity. Initially, a broad spectrum antibiotic may be prescribed, as well as decongestant nose drops (see page 64). If this does not bring about a resolution of the infection, surgery will be necessary. This involves cracking a hole in the bone between the lacrimal fossa and the nasal cavity. The aim is to affect a junction between the lacrimal fossa and the nasal mucosa. Closure of this junction is not infrequent as the body does not tolerate abnormal apertures.

Trauma

Rupture of the canaliculus in the lower lid is a common windscreen injury, possibly less common now that seatbelts are obligatory. Failure to secure the torn ends within 24 hours of injury raises the risk of an intractable watering that may well defeat the ingenuity of the surgeon, the tolerance of the patient and may also produce a mountain of legal and insurance reports.

Eight
The red eye

Introduction

Before we can call an eye abnormal and red, we must define what we mean by normal and white. Such a definition is based on the appearances of the conjunctiva and these vary with their position. To begin with, the sclera is seen as eggshell white through translucent vascular conjunctiva. As the conjunctiva folds away into the fornix, the blood vessels begin to dominate as the sclera becomes less apparent, and the conjunctiva becomes pinker and pinker until on the surface of the eyelid, it is almost red.

There are three major 'red eyes'—keratitis, iritis and acute glaucoma. They dilate vessels within the eye, but only those around the corneoscleral limbus are readily visible. Thus inflammation around the edge of the cornea is a warning sign of an eye in serious danger. All other red eyes, no matter what their cause, are less red beside the cornea than they are away from it.

There is only one decision therefore which has to be made about a red eye. Is it one of the major three or not? If it is, then the examination ritual will indicate which of the major three it is every time.

Keratitis

In practical terms, any breach of the corneal epithelium is, or may lead to keratitis. The breach may be traumatic or the results of infection by micro-organisms or irritation by chemicals (Fig. 8.1).

Examination and clinical features

In addition to pain, redness and watering, the patient will admit to loss of central vision. The reduction of central vision will depend on the actual position of the ulcer. The visual field will be unaffected. Corneal lustre will be lost and the exact area of deficient

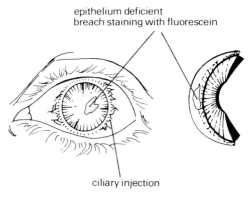

epithelium deficient
breach staining with fluorescein

ciliary injection

Fig. 8.1 Keratitis. One of the three major red eyes; the cornea stains with fluorescein, and is seen more clearly when brought close with a small convex lens.

epithelium can be demonstrated by instilling one or more drops of sodium fluorescein. A normal pupil is common unless an incidental iritis has already stuck it to the lens. The anterior chamber of both eyes will be deep (eclipse test).

Treatment

The aim of treatment is to reverse the ill effects of the cause. Should infection predominate, then it must be vigorously treated with intensive topical and possibly systemic antibiotics. An associated iritis requires dilatation of the pupil with topical atropine, for reasons that have already been explained. It might even require topical corticosteroids. In the acute stage the exquisite pain will defeat standard analgesics, and indeed opiates may well be the only source of relief.

The broken epithelium frequently heals best behind eyelids closed either with adhesive tape or with frank stitching (tarsorrhaphy). Finally once all has settled, if the patient is dissatisfied with the scarred cornea, then a corneal graft could well be indicated.

Iritis

Clinical features

The redness may be very much the same as in keratitis, but the pain may be rather less. In addition, inflammatory debris exuding into the aqueous and vitreous will dance across the visual line as floaters.

Central vision can be anything from normal downwards, depending on previous damage or the severity of the present attack. The field is generally unaffected.

The corneal surface glistens normally, but deposits of inflammatory material (keratic precipitates) may be seen on the deep surface of the cornea with a magnifying lens (Fig. 8.2).

A spastic pupil is common because of irritation of the iris sphincter. Also, previous adhesions may have stuck the iris down irregularly. The anterior chamber in both eyes has no reason to be shallow. The management has already been described as an example of treatment principles (Ch. 6).

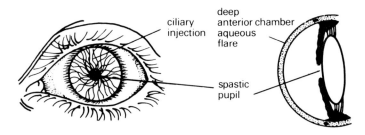

Fig. 8.2 Iritis. One of the three major red eyes; the cornea is normal and the pupil possibly spastic; flare and keratic precipitates are more obvious when brought close with a small convex lens.

Acute glaucoma

Clinical features

The evident distress of the patient will cut short the tell-tale story of haloes, frontal headache and transient attacks of blurred vision in the evening. Central vision will be severely affected though the patient may be too distressed to co-operate in estimating the visual field.

Examination of the eye reveals an oedematous cornea which obscures the deeper signs (Fig. 8.3). The pupil, which can be seen through the cornea, will be fixed and dilated. The anterior chamber will be shallow (eclipse test). If it is obscured by the cornea, then there is always the fellow eye to look at. The affected eye will be rock hard and acutely tender. The treatment and nursing care are described in a later chapter on glaucoma.

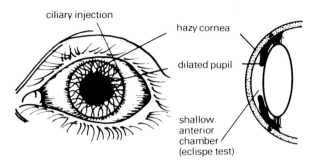

ciliary injection

hazy cornea

dilated pupil

shallow
anterior
chamber
(eclispe test)

Fig. 8.3 Acute glaucoma. One of the three major red eyes; the cornea is hazy, the pupil fixed and dilated, the anterior chamber shallow on both sides (Eclipse test).

Discussion

Once we can recognise when an eye is inflamed by one of the major three we will also be in a position to recognise when it is not. *As a general rule the less dangerous a red eye might be the more alarming it will appear.*

Subconjunctival haemorrhage and conjunctivitis can both appear frightful, and if the cardinal signs of the cornea and the pupil and the depth between them are neglected in favour of the overall impression, then they may be given a significance greater than they deserve. They may even give a spurious attraction to the alternative, but lethal, diagnosis by ordeal of inflamed eyes into those that seem to improve with corticosteroids and those that do not.

Of the three major causes of a red eye, keratitis has signs in the cornea; acute glaucoma has signs in the cornea, anterior chamber depth and the pupil; iritis may only have inflammation around the cornea to mark it off from the other causes of red eye. The special rule is to use the same examination ritual every time, and not to suspend clinical judgement just because the redness happens to be in the eye and not somewhere else.

Nine
Cataract

The lens has one basic response to insult—it becomes opaque. Different degrees of disturbance cause different degrees of opacity, but whatever their degree we call them all cataract, preferably softening the word, for most people have a mortal dread of the name.

Causes of cataract

There are many causes of cataract. An example of a systemic disorder is rubella infection during the first trimester of pregnancy. Cataracts may be familial, traumatic, inflammatory or metabolic, e.g. diabetes mellitus. Ionising radiation must also be regarded as harmful. Prolonged exposure to infra-red light produces cataract at an early age in the tropics, and fat dogs whose only exercise is to blink their eyelids from time to time before a grate blazing with logs suffer the same condition. However, the commonest cause is (ageing) senility and it may be thought of as part of the same process that turns the hair grey.

Examination and clinical features

The primary complaint is visual loss and examination will reveal disturbance in central vision. The cornea will be clear and the pupil will react normally to light. The anterior chamber depth can be gauged using the eclipse test and will usually be normal. The intra-ocular pressure need not be raised just because the patient has a cataract—but it may be raised because the patient is old enough to have a cataract *and* chronic glaucoma. The cataract can be seen as an opacity against the red reflex coming from the back of the eye, and is best seen through a dilated pupil (Figs. 9.1 and 9.2).

Treatment and nursing care

It is impossible to reduce less opacities with medication of any sort.

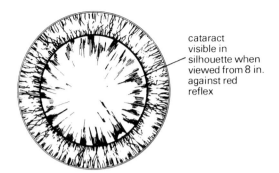

Fig. 9.1 Cataract. Discovered by the technique shown in Figure 9.2.

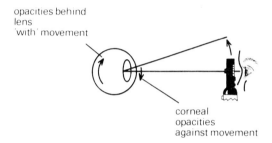

Fig. 9.2 How to detect opacities through the dilated pupil against the red reflex.

This has not stopped unscrupulous charlatans from promising miracles with vegetable diets and drugs of an organic origin and long walks through the Swiss mountains.

However, it is possible to improve the vision on a temporary basis by dilating the pupil with atropine drops. This allows the patient to look around the cataract, and, if glasses tinted with sodium yellow are used, it may allow light to enter the eye without dazzle. In addition it has the quality of making every day seem bathed in sunshine—a remarkable and precious attribute in a British January.

The only real treatment is surgery, but it is best to delay the operation until the patient can no longer function happily in his own environment. This is a field where many changes are taking place, but with many variations on an essential theme which is to remove the opaque lens from its position behind the iris.

Operation

A 180° incision is made around the cornea and the lens is removed—commonly with a freezing probe (Fig. 9.3).

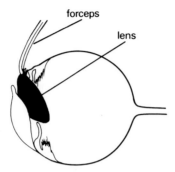

Fig. 9.3 Cataract extraction. There are many similarities between obstetrics and ophthalmology, not least the delivery of a reluctant object through an orifice that seems ridiciulously small until the last moment.

Pre-operative care

The patient will usually be admitted the day before surgery. In some units, where surgery is done on a day-care basis, the patient will be screened and his history recorded before he comes to the centre, often at the out-patient department. The pre-operative care is, however, similar, regardless of whether the patient is a day case or an in-patient.

A careful nursing history is taken and an explanation of what is to happen is given to the patient. Many of the patients will be elderly and will have many concurrent health problems such as diabetes and hypertension. All medications for such disorders are given as per usual unless prescribed otherwise. All the normal pre-operative care is required. A mild sedative may be prescribed the night before to ensure a good night's sleep. Some doctors prescribe antibiotic drops such as chloramphenicol. The doctor will examine the patient carefully to ensure that he is clear of infection and that the tear ducts are patent. Conjunctival swabs may be taken for culture and sensitivity.

On the morning of the operation the patient is dressed in a loose-fitting gown. The eyelashes are trimmed using scissors smeared in petroleum jelly. This prevents eyelashes falling into the wound and causing infection. (They grow back in about 3 weeks.) A mydriatic such as cyclopentolate 1% is given to dilate the pupil. Local anaesthetic drops may also be prescribed for instillation immediately prior to surgery, the main anaesthetic effect being achieved by retrobulbar and facial nerve injections of lignocaine 2% and adrenaline. Some patients are given a general anaesthetic and must be prepared accordingly.

Post-operative care

The eye is usually covered with a pad. The patient is nursed in bed, well supported by pillows, or he may be allowed to sit in a comfortable chair. If all is well he can then be given a cup of tea and reassured that a nurse will always be close by if he requires any assistance. Any pain is treated with soluble codeine or, if it is more severe, with dihydrocodeine. Deep breathing should be encouraged, though coughing should be discouraged as this may cause an increase in the intra-ocular pressure, as may vomiting. If either condition is present, it should be reported to the doctor who can then prescribe appropriate medication.

The patient should manage a cup of tea quite soon after the operation and he can usually manage a normal diet. Hard or chewy foods should be avoided and false teeth, if used, should be worn. The patient may often be allowed up by the evening and in the case of day patients, be ready for discharge. The patient must be informed not to touch or press his eye. He should avoid bending over, for example to pick something up. Any tendency to constipation should be alleviated by the judicious use of dietary fibre, a bulking agent or laxative. Straining at stool leads to a marked rise in intracranial pressure which in turn causes a rise in intra-ocular pressure.

The first dressing is done usually four to five hours post-operation. The eye pad is removed and the eye is then bathed with sterile normal saline. Eye drops are instilled as prescribed. Some surgeons like to keep the eye covered by a pad or shield for up to a week. Other surgeons prescribe dark glasses or appropriate aphakic glasses which are worn constantly day and night, except when drops are being instilled. Antibiotics and/or steroid drops are often prescribed as well as a mydriatic/cycloplegic. Patients must be warned that visual distortion is always present following the operation, especially when aphakic glasses are worn, and that it will take some time to get used to them. They must be told not to drive as both visual field and depth of vision are seriously distorted.

Before discharge the patient should be given instructions on the self-administration of eye drops if these are prescribed (see p. 193). It may be necessary to instruct a relative on how to do this. Information should also be given on what to do if any problems arise, and arrangements should be made for follow-up visits.

Discussion

The removal of the lens is the removal of a vital element of the optical arrangement of the eye and this has to be corrected.

The most frequent and the most unpleasant correction is a thick pair of spectacles which magnify the image and minify the field. This produces a ghastly jack-in-the-box effect where images suddenly vanish and just as suddenly reappear. Not infrequently the older age group fail to tolerate this at all. The next step is to apply a contact lens which is anatomically nearer the position of the removed cataract. Not everyone can wear a contact lens and even fewer people can manipulate its positioning and removal. For this reason, particularly in the elderly, long-wear contact lenses have been developed, and of course these must allow unhampered passage of oxygen to the cornea.

Given these innate difficulties it is not surprising that strenuous attempts have been made to improve upon that situation. In recent years an increasing number of cataracts have been replaced by a Perspex lens within the eye itself.

That intra-ocular perspex might be tolerated indefinitely became evident during the last war when pilots retained functioning eyes despite the presence of windscreen fragments within. From this observation has grown a huge market for intra-ocular lenses. Not so long ago the question used to be: why an intra-ocular lens? Now it tends to be, why not?

Ten
The glaucomas

Definition

Glaucoma can be defined as any state where the intra-ocular pressure rises above what we accept as normal. It will result from any form of blockage to the aqueous circulation at any point in its journey from the ciliary body through the pupil to the meshwork of the drainage angle of the anterior chamber.

Causes

If the cause is known, for example iritic adhesions at the pupil, we call it glaucoma secondary to iritis. If due to a narrow angle, we call it closed angle or acute glaucoma. If due to no recognisable cause then, with a fine sense of irony and a certain degree of effrontery, we call it glaucoma simplex.

By an unfortunate mischance, the term glaucoma derives from the Greek word for cataract. An eye used to be described as glaucous when advancing cataract gave the lens that greenish tinge allegedly associated with poor vision.

In more rugged times when many eyes ended up blind and green from as many causes, the term glaucoma was applied to all of them. However, advancing knowledge has now renamed most of them according to their special pathology, but not always as helpfully as we might wish. Glaucoma which does not turn the eye green, has retained the term glaucoma, whilst the original condition which actually did is now called cataract. Alas!

Acute glaucoma (closed angle)

The popular misconception of acute glaucoma is that it is chronic glaucoma with a degree of urgency and haloes. Unfortunately this is not the case. There is no connection in any way between the two conditions, unless someone is unfortunate enough to have both.

Acute glaucoma is not so much a disease as a shape. It occurs in the long sighted eye, with an anterior chamber too shallow for safe dilatation of the pupil. The advance of middle age exaggerates this shallowness by a forward movement of the iris lens diaphragm.

Extreme long sight has two further associates—thick glasses that obscure distanct objects to all but those for whom they were prescribed, and not infrequently a convergent squint dating from childhood.

Dilatation of the pupil, however, is not the whole story. Active impulses of the sympathetic innervated radial dilating fibres, drag the iris back against the lens, blocking the flow of aqueous through the pupil. The aqueous, failing to pass the pupil, pushes the peripheral iris against the cornea with sudden obstruction to the outflow.

This *coup de grâce* does not come out of the blue. Rather does it come out of a collection of colours known as haloes. Transient attacks of acute glaucoma raise the pressure of the eyeball and force fluid into the cornea. Not unnaturally pain in the adjacent forehead follows the first, whilst blurred vision follows the second. Haloes also follow the second because the corneal oedema breaks the light into the colours of the spectrum, producing the colours of a rainbow in the form of a ring—round because the cornea is round.

The anticipation of likely victims, and the prevention of such tragic attacks, is the third major aim of ophthalmic examination. The condition is so easy to treat before it has happened that to leave it to happen borders on negligence.

Treatment and nursing care

Before it has happened, the treatment is surgical—an irridectomy cut on the periphery of the iris, bypassing any resistance at the pupil.

However, when the attack has happened we have an ocular emergency. The patient is in pain, the vision is hazy, in both central and field vision. The cornea is hazy. The pupil if seen through the hazy cornea, is fixed and dilated. The anterior chamber is seen through the hazy cornea as shallow. If it cannot be seen then the same shape might be demonstrated in the fellow eye. What the actual treatment is can be worked out from what we actually know. If the pressure is raised it must be brought down. The drugs used to reduce the intra-ocular pressure are acetazolamide (Ch. 15), which can be given orally or by injection, and pilocarpine, which is used topically. Pilocarpine is a sympathomimetic agent which constricts the pupil (Fig. 10.1). It has to be poured onto the eye

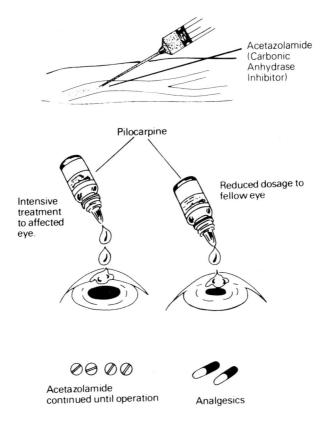

Fig. 10.1 Acute glaucoma therapy.

intensively to achieve this. If the pressure can be broken quickly, then surgery can be a matter of convenience. If the attack cannot be broken then a hole has to be cut in the eye to allow aqueous to drain permanently into the subconjunctival space (Fig. 10.2).

Chronic glaucoma

This is a most sinister and tragic cause of blindness: sinister because it is usually symptomless until gross field loss can no longer be ignored, and tragic because it could have been arrested in the first place. If patients have heard at all about glaucoma, it will be the acute painful variety. Otherwise they ascribe any visual loss to cataract, which they have all heard about and which they all usually get wrong as well.

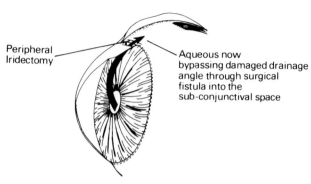

Peripheral Iridectomy

Aqueous now bypassing damaged drainage angle through surgical fistula into the sub-conjunctival space

Fig. 10.2 Peripheral irridectomy.

In normal circumstances there is a happy balance between the pressure of the eyeball and the pressure of blood supplying the optic nerve head.

However in glaucoma this balance is upset, and a battle develops in its place between the pressure of blood trying to stop it. If the intra-ocular pressure wins then the capillary closure begins to starve the peripheral retina.

The disease is diagnosed, not because patients complain about anything (Fig. 10.3), but because they fear that they may be harbouring something of which they are totally unaware.

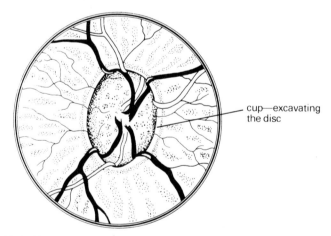

cup—excavating the disc

Fig. 10.3 Glaucoma. A grossly cupped optic disc—the tragic result of not having the eyes examined until after something goes wrong—or of incompetent examination before something has gone wrong—and occasionally after. A safe eye is one that does not harbour an undiagnosed glaucoma.

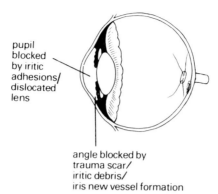

pupil
blocked
by iritic
adhesions/
dislocated
lens

angle blocked by
trauma scar/
iritic debris/
iris new vessel formation

Fig. 10.4 Secondary glaucoma. The circulation of aqueous may be obstructed at many points, by many conditions. The condition may be obvious; the aqueous obstruction may not. Once again the patient does not recognise that the field is going until it is gone.

Treatment aims to reduce the intra-ocular pressure. The various drugs used to do this are described in Chapter 16. If all medical measures fail then surgery is required.

The surgeon aims to drain off aqueous through a permanent fistula into the subconjunctival space. The body does not approve of such unnatural channels and may close them off with fibrous tissue, especially in younger patients.

Secondary glaucoma

When the intra-ocular pressure rises in response to any other recognisable agency we use the term secondary glaucoma. Strictly speaking all glaucomas are secondary to something! It is just that in chronic simple glaucoma we do not yet know to what. Because closed angle glaucoma is always due to the same thing, it has been granted a title in its own right (Fig. 10.4).

Eleven

Squints

The eyes normally move together in parallel to extend that range of vision which is already made available by the swivelling and nodding action of the head and neck. They can also move against each other out of parallel when they converge to focus on a near object—a reflex not uncommonly weakened when the shocks of existence, either physical or spiritual, become too much to bear.

Critical distinction

Squinting eyes fall naturally into two groups:
1. those without binocular vision,
2. those with binocular vision.

The distinction is critical. In the first group, because the eyes cannot work together they work separately. Because they are pointing in different directions they therefore cannot work at the same time. The result is the alternating use of either eye, or the habitual use of one eye, while the other lapses into a state of lazy amblyopia (absence of central vision in the presence of a normal eye).

The second group do work together, because the brain has learned to interpret their simultaneous flow of similar images (Fig. 11.1). Separation of these eyes, classically by a paralysed muscle, will produce a simultaneous flow of wholly dissimilar images. Each eye will continue to see but not the same thing, and the result is a bitter complaint of double vision. The latter is almost always due to a paralysed muscle.

Eyes without binocular vision

As a squint can generally only be demonstrated by someone who is used to demonstrating it, most squints that come our way are because parents or relatives imagine that there is something the

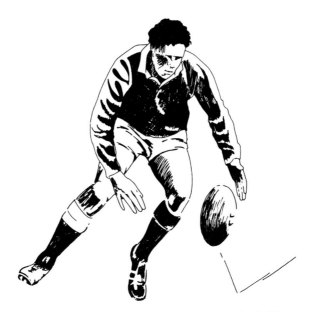

Fig. 11.1 Binocular vision. To catch a bouncing rugby ball is one of its supreme tests. If binocular vision is present the classic childhood squint is not; its presence can be proved.

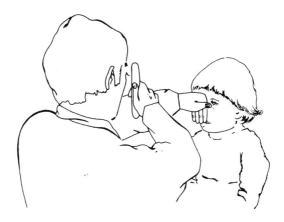

Fig. 11.2 The cover test.

matter with the child's eyes, although they are not quite sure exactly what (Fig. 11.2 and Fig. 11.3). The essential step is to demonstrate the presence of macular function in each eye separately. This is not perhaps as difficult as might be thought in a 3-

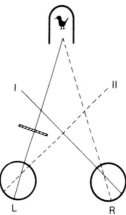

Position I
L eye fixing
R eye convergent at a particular angle.
Position II
L eye covered
R eye now moved out to fix
L eye follows it in like the reins of a horse. *The angle of squint remains unchanged.*

Fig. 11.3 What the cover test reveals.

year old. Little sticks are available with pictures of teddy bears and houses which correspond, as near as makes no difference, to the smallest reading print. If each eye separately can make out this difference, then at least that means that macular vision is functioning. If there is a squint, and there may still be, then at least the major part of treatment is unnecessary.

The major part of treatment, of course, is to establish central vision. The best available chance is between the age of 6 months and 6 years, with the chance progressively diminishing as the years progress. However, the chances really do not start until the age of 2, as most children below that age cannot really co-operate.

The child is handed over to orthoptists who are well practised in wheedling information out of truculent 3-year olds. If the central vision of one eye can be reduced, even with appropriate glasses, then the orthoptists will set out on a course of patching. This involves occlusion of the good eye during the waking hours for something like a month at a time to force the poorer eye to drive its functional pathway through to the brain.

Although explanations may be conducted amidst smiling good-will, it is the mother who has to deal with all the tantrums and defiance during the period of occlusion. It is vital that it is carried out ruthlessly by a combination of cajolery and resistance to tearful promises of good behaviour tomorrow, if only the patch can come off today.

The aim of treatment is to establish equal macular function. Once the child is capable of fixing alternately with either eye, the visual pathways have been established.

Surgery

Surgery is usually for cosmetic reasons and is usually the last step in the line of treatment. In some countries where such a service is not readily available or welcomed, an imposing squint may be considered a token of military genius, or at least a delivery system for evil rays. Such prized qualities, often leading to tribal leadership, will not be lightly exchanged for a comely appearance.

However, in most parts of the world cosmetic appearance is paramount and the best time is before the child goes to school, when his fellows' facility for wounding nicknames will be frustrated. Since this child does not have binocular vision, the eyes once straightened may finally diverge, because the orbits point outwards anyway. Such divergence can of course be reversed by further surgery some years later still.

Nursing aspects of squint surgery

Pre-operative preparation

Most surgery for squint is done on children. The child is admitted to hospital on the morning of the operation or on the previous day. All explanation should be given in terms the child can understand. Hospitalisation is a frightening experience for the child and separation from the mother will make the child cry. Whenever possible one nurse should have responsibility for the preparation of the child for surgery as children respond best to being cared for by one individual. Regression, for example bedwetting and the development of other nervous habits, may occur. Most operations are done under general anaesthesia and the child requires all the normal preoperative care. It is important that they have had nothing to eat or drink since midnight of the previous evening. In the case of day patients this fact must be clearly established. Young children do not understand why they must not eat or drink and may not comply, so they must be observed very carefully. A premedication will be prescribed depending on the anaesthetist's/surgeon's preference (see section on pre-operative care). Some doctors also prescribe antibiotic drops prior to surgery to remove as many pathogens from the conjunctiva as possible.

Post-operative care

On return to the ward the child will require all the usual post-operative care. The child may or may not be wearing an eyepatch, depending on the surgeon's directions. Discharge is usually minimal. Some doctors prescribe an antibiotic eye drop or steroid several times a day for the first week to relieve inflammation. The antibiotic may also be prescribed as an ointment which has a soothing effect. Warm compresses can also be used to relieve pain. If pain is persistent analgesics will be required. The child should be instructed not to rub or press his eye as this will make it sore. The child will have some degree of visual disability so that nursing care should be geared to this. Stay in hospital is usually short, and treatment, such as eyepatching and drops, must be continued at home. A careful explanation of their use should be given to the parents. They may well be alarmed when they see the eye red and inflamed and should be reassured this will subside in a week or so, provided they administer the drops as instructed. Parents need to be instructed in maintaining a safe environment for the child whilst the eyepatch is being worn, and also about follow-up visits and what to do if the redness and discomfort do not settle in a few days. The eyepatch reduces the annoyance of natural and artificial light which may lead to increased redness, burning and tearing, tempting the patient to rub or touch the eye and so making the condition worse and increasing the risk of introducing infection. If there is doubt about the parents' ability to care adequately for the child at home during this period, arrangements should be made for a community nurse to call or the child may have to be detained for a few days longer in hospital.

The post-operative care of adults following correction of squint is essentially the same as described above: a liberal regime being adopted for example, up to the toilet in the evening and a return to normal diet established as soon as the patient feels up to it. Patients can read and watch television if they wish and should be fit for work in about a week.

Amblyopia

To complete our list of popular misconceptions, it is commonly believed that a lazy eye (amblyopic) must be a squinting eye. Now for reasons which should now be apparent, while most squinting eyes may become lazy, not all lazy eyes squint. They may be straight, but deprived of macular stimulation by anything that interferes with the fixing mechanism—from ptosis (a dropped eyelid) through congenital cataract to glasses unworn when glasses should be worn.

Eyes with binocular function

Any disease from the brain stem to the orbit can cause a muscle to malfunction. The commonest cause is a head injury, which may produce anything from simple bruising to total destruction of the brain.

Intracranial lesions, such as an aneurysm or a brain tumour, are more common in the younger age groups, while diabetes, hypertension and arteriosclerosis are associated with the older age groups.

Fluctuating double vision, worsening towards the end of the day, is almost diagnostic of myasthenia gravis, whilst a muscle palsy as part of an unconnected catalogue of signs must raise the spectre of multiple sclerosis.

Twelve
Systemic disorders which affect eyes

Diabetes

Diabetes is one of the most common causes of blindness in the West today. In the young, its major complication—retinopathy—begins some 15 years after the onset of the disease, but there is no doubt that this time lapse can be extended by careful diabetic control.

Maturity onset diabetics, on the contrary, may be quite unaware of their metabolic problems until a sudden haemorrhage into the vitreous initiates a series of medical investigations that seem bafflingly remote from the eye.

Diabetes affects small blood vessels all over the body, but only in the eye can these changes be seen. These blood vessels tend to leak their contents into the tissues. Fat depositing in the macula, damages irrevocably central vision. Blood leaking out into and beyond the retina can produce even more dramatic loss of both central and field vision (Fig. 12.1 and Fig. 12.2).

Although the vessels freely leak their content into the tissues, they are not so good at allowing the blood to arrive where it belongs

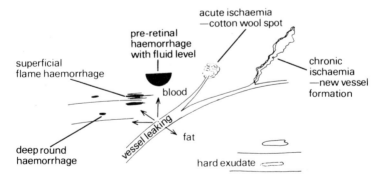

Fig. 12.1 Diabetic micro-angiopathy. The process behind what we call diabetic retinopathy.

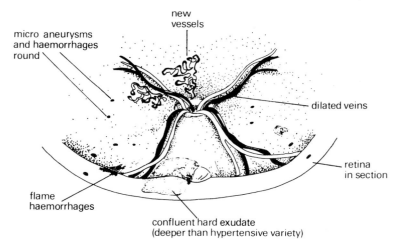

micro aneurysms
and haemorrhages
round

new
vessels

dilated veins

retina
in section

flame
haemorrhages

confluent hard exudate
(deeper than hypertensive variety)

Fig. 12.2 Diabetic retinopathy. Related to duration and poor control.

naturally. Sudden failure of blood flow can produce acute infarction of the retina. More leisurely blockage causes hypoxia. Poorly-fed retinal tissue then in search of more oxygen creates new blood vessels in the hope of supplying this want. However, although the retina may get oxygen, the vitreous gets blood, because these vessels have a tendency to spontaneous rupture—a tendency encouraged by high blood pressure. There then starts a cycle of new blood vessel formation, followed by bleeding into the vitreous, followed by fibrosis and traction retinal detachment. This cycle can lead to total blindness.

Treatment

The best treatment is prevent, but once the eye has demonstrated an oxygen requirement beyond the level of oxygen availability, the only possible treatment is to reduce the oxygen requirements.

This is produced by inflicting a series of laser burns over the entire retina. Once the requirement level equals the availability level, then the stimulus to these vascular catastrophes is removed (Fig. 12.3).

Hypertension

The response of the eye to hypertension, like so much else, can be made incomprehensible if so desired, over several chapters. Yet

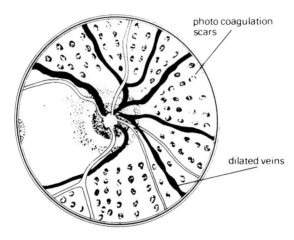

Fig. 12.3 Diabetic retinopathy treated with the argon laser. An iatrogenic healed chorioretinitis.

predictably, perhaps, the whole matter can be reduced to a few simple elements:

1. the state of the blood vessels
2. the rate of hypertensive change
3. the extent of hypertensive change.

   In youth the retinal vessels are well endowed with elastic tissue and the arterioles also with muscle. As age advances, the elasticity gives way to fibrous tissue which protects the vessels somewhat against rises in blood pressure. A sudden increase in the blood pressure would clearly have a more devastating effect on the unprepared eye of childhood; a more gradual and a more moderate increase may have little effect on the old eye and on the young eye it may accelerate ageing changes. Whatever the age of the patient, when the blood pressure does rise above what is medically accepted as normal, there is a further change within the blood vessels which make them less capable of carrying out their function as a carrier of blood to essential tissues.

Effects of hyp rtension

All the calamities associated with hypertension over the rest of the body can occur in the eye.

1. Bleeding may occur underneath the conjunctiva, where it is of no significance unless it is ignored and is a sign of more potentially serious bleeding elsewhere.

2. Bleeding into the vitreous is of course a catastrophe which obscures vision and which may take its time to clear, if it ever does.
3. Blockage of the central retinal artery can of course produce a 'stroke' within the eye and totally destroy the retina's capacity for light perception.
4. Blockage of a vein, on the other hand, although also devastating, does not totally destroy vision.
5. Local changes within the retina itself can of course damage the area of central vision and this is a not uncommon presenting symptom of hypertension.

Treatment

There are one or two simple principles. Young patients may have some recognisable cause for their hypertension, which can be removed with total recovery.

The problem starts in the elderly, who may well be used to their level of blood pressure, where overkeen reduction might turn a simple ophthalmoscopic observation into a genuine disability. The presence of even one cotton wool spot means the vascular tree is already beyond repair. In general terms, the more pronounced the arterio-venous crossing change the less likely is treatment to be successful.

It is too late to remove macular exudates once they have formed. Their existence should be forestalled.

The ophthalmologist can do little to treat any resultant visual loss. All he can do is warn the physician what his findings imply.

The nursing care aspects of the diabetic and hypertensive patient can be found in any good medical nursing text and will not be elaborated on here.

Thirteen
Disorders of the retina

Retinal detachment

A retinal detachment is not really a detachment at all, but a separation of two distinct retinal layers. However the term detachment, lingering on from the pioneering days of ophthalmology, has lingered too long to tolerate substitution. The neuro-retina and the pigment retina normally give up their independent existence to fuse into a composite epithelium, which secretes aqueous from a deep surface of the ciliary body.

The transfusion from two layers to one takes place in a scalloped line, more remembered for its quaint name—ora serrata—than for its actual position. Marking the anterior limit of the functioning retina this ora serrata lies deep to a line connecting the insertions of the four rectus muscles (Fig. 13.1). Any injury perforating the globe behind this line will certainly perforate the retina as well, and as certainly cause it to detach.

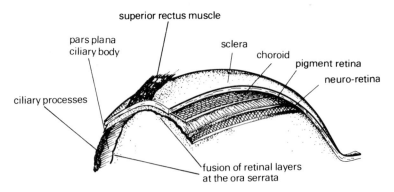

Fig. 13.1 The ocular layers. The two retinal layers fuse at the ora serrata, posterior to which separation of one retina from the other is called a retinal detachment. The rectus insertions are at the scleral landmark of the ora serrata.

The two layers are adherent also at the optic nerve head, but a potential space remains between them everywhere else. When we talk of a retinal detachment we mean that a potentially mobile neuro-retina has for some reason abandoned its natural position of contact with the outer pigment retina.

Pathology and clinical features

The commonest cause of a retinal detachment is a break in the retina, through which passes liquified vitreous which separates the neural layer from the pigment layer. Once separated, this neural layer begins to starve and if separated long enough will starve to death, becoming in the process so fibrotic that mechanical replacement would be impossible even if enough functioning retina remained to justify the attempt.

Abnormal adhesions of the vitreous to the retina facilitates the formation of retinal breaks. Repetitive traction on this adhesion will stimulate the retina into the only response left available by its high degree of specialisation—light flashing. As the retina tears, the flashing lights stop, though rupture of a blood vessel may fill the vitreous cavity with blood and the visual field with a sudden shower of floaters. There is no pain, only panic.

Patients at risk

Myopia. Myopic retinae, not sufficient in these large eyes to cover all the areas that the retina should cover, are much more liable to perforate and hence to detach than are those of normal eyes.

Cataract removal. Removal of a cataract leaves a space into which the vitreous advances pulling on its normal attachment at the ora serrata.

Trauma. Trauma can of course rip the retina in any position; congenital defects in development can produce the same effect without injury.

Treatment and nursing care

The aim of surgery is to find the retinal break and this can only be done satisfactorily with the indirect ophthalmoscope because the view with the direct ophthalmoscope fails to reach anterior to the equator.

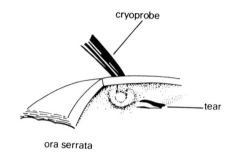

Fig. 13.2 Freezing all the layers of the eye around a retinal tear.

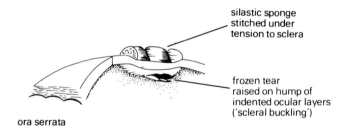

Fig. 13.3 One way to seal a retinal tear.

Inflammation is then induced around the break from outside the eye; this is currently done by use of a freezing pencil (Fig. 13.2). The retinal layers around the break are then held watertight until the inflammation forms a scar, which should also be watertight.

Because of the dangers of persisting traction on the retina which may pull the tear open again, it is customary to reduce the volume of the eye by some form of scleral buckling. This involves the stitching of inert materials, such as silicone rubber or silastic sponge on to the sclera, to push the ocular layer inwards (Fig. 13.3), or injection of air into the vitreous to float the retinal tear upwards. The success rate should be in the order of 95% (Fig. 13.4).

Although the majority of detachments are produced by retinal tears, occasionally a tumour of the choroid, whether primary or secondary, may produce an appearance not dissimilar to the casual observer.

Pre-operative care

The patient will usually, though not always, be admitted on the day the surgeon has made the diagnosis. These patients are always very

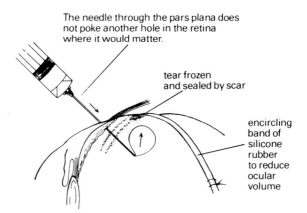

The needle through the pars plana does
not poke another hole in the retina
where it would matter.

tear frozen
and sealed by scar

encircling
band of
silicone
rubber
to reduce
ocular
volume

Fig. 13.4 Another way to seal a retinal tear.

anxious, having just experienced some rapid loss of vision. Blindness
or the fear of losing sight seems very real, given the usually sudden
onset of the condition. Nurses can do much to allay apprehension by
reinforcing the possibility of a favourable outcome. It is, of course,
the surgeon's responsibility to reassure the patient regarding the
prognosis.

If this is not good, the nurses should be informed so that
consistent information is given. Because the patient is anxious he
will often ask the same question over and over again, as he finds
it difficult to comprehend what is happening to him and is, perhaps,
also hoping for a more favourable report. Many problems arise
through inadequate communications. With a little thought, the
patient's experience can be made at least more tolerable.

In former days retinal surgery induced a violent inflammation in
the coats of the eye in the quadrant of the retinal break. Prolonged
bed rest with the head immobilised between sandbags and a diet
of gruel was considered necessary to give the retina some chance
of settling and sticking. It did not always stick, but the instinctive
call for bed rest has remained, even to this day.

Because vision is usually restricted, the patient must take care
not to bump into or trip over anything as this may lead to further
damage. The pupil is dilated to permit easier examination of the
retina at any time and to prevent iritis.

The patient requires all the usual pre-operative care. Eye drops—
mydriatrics, cycloplegics and antibiotics—are administered as
prescribed. The eyelashes are trimmed. The hair should be gently
shampooed the day before surgery; the nurse take care not to let
the patient bend forwards over the sink. Hair washing before the

operation aids patient comfort as this will not be permitted very often for up to a week after the operation. The patient should be told that his eye may be discoloured and swollen, depending on the procedure used. There is no single modality which is applied in the care of patients with retinal detachments. Much depends on the surgeon's preference.

The post-operative care is essentially the same as that following cataract removal. The patient may have one or both eyes patched, depending on the surgeon's directions. It is usual for the eye which has been treated to be patched. There is nothing to recommend the patching of both eyes. If both eyes are covered, safety precautions are essential.

Dilatation of the pupil is maintained by the use of mydriatic/cycloplegic agents. In addition, steroid drops are usually given to reduce inflammation. The eyelids on some occasions may be very swollen, depending on the amount of manipulation required during surgery. The amount of swelling and bruising is more extensive when 'scleral buckling' has been done, as the eyelids have to be manipulated to gain access.

The patient should be reassured that this is self-limiting. If the eyelids are stuck together on removal of the patch the discharge is removed using sterile saline or water. Cold compresses several times per day may be ordered to reduce swelling and ecchymosis.

Activity orders vary. Prolonged bed rest is unnecessary and most patients will be allowed up to the bathroom the first day, after which a fairly liberal routine is allowed. Activity actually helps the retina to stick.

Some patients experience pain or discomfort in the operated eye. Analgesia, prescribed according to the severity of pain, should be given. Any nausea or vomiting can be relieved if an appropriate antiemetic is used.

On some occasions the surgeon will inject air as mentioned above. The patient has to be positioned carefully so that when the air rises it will mechanically press against the area which needs to be flattened. The surgeon will indicate the exact position of head placement. It is important that this position is maintained for the time specified. Since the air moves to the highest part of the globe it may, for example, escape into the anterior chamber in an aphakic patient who lies supine.

Deep breathing is encouraged but coughing must be avoided, if possible, to reduce the risk of raising the intra-ocular pressure. Reading is positively discouraged, though watching television at a moderate distance may be permitted if the patient uses the untreated eye. Handwork may be allowed, if it does not cause discomfort.

Great care must be taken to prevent infection as the risk of this is heightened because of the swollen eyelids and discharge. All patients are extremely anxious and require reassurance. As sight cannot be guaranteed it is a worrying time for the patient and his family.

In caring for the patient the nurse should observe for any increase in swelling or discharge. Any complaints of pain, nausea, vomiting or haloes should be reported to the doctor. These signs and symptoms may be evidence of infection or glaucoma.

Prior to discharge the patient should be given instructions on what he should avoid doing. This includes reading, lifting heavy objects, bending the head below waist level, straining of any kind especially as a result of constipation. Hair should be washed preferably in the shower to avoid bending, or by a hairdresser with the head back. It is best to watch television from a distance to avoid discomfort. The wearing of dark glasses may add to patient comfort, by reducing the annoyance of both natural and artificial light. Driving is prohibited.

Instructions are given to the patient regarding instillation of drops and on how to clean round the eyes using sterile cotton or gauze sponges moistened in sterile saline. Details are given regarding follow-up visits and what to do if the patient's vision deteriorates or other complications develop.

Fourteen

Injuries to the eye and related structures

Injuries, no matter where they strike the body, have two important aspects. The first and obvious one is the instant damage they cause. The second is the possible long-term complication, either at the site of injury or at a more distant site.

Apart from a few well-defined conditions demanding urgent specialist attention, most lacerations around the eye are ocular only because they happen to be in that area.

Injuries become 'specialist ocular' in four main categories, and the only equipment necessary to evaluate the damage is a good torch, whilst the other eye may serve as a normal control.

Intra-ocular foreign body

In any violence involving the eye, a foreign body within the globe should always be suspected (Fig. 14.1). Close examination of the eyeball may show an entry point—iris distortion being a helpful guide. But a fragment entering the limbus could leave the eye looking entirely normal until its ill effects become obvious some time later. Most foreign bodies are radio-opaque and this quality should be used when making a diagnosis.

If the foreign body has perforated the lens, then a cataract will almost certainly follow. If it has perforated the retina, then a detachment will follow. If it is left inside the eye, then its chemical constituents will dissolve in the ocular fluids, destroying the eye in the process.

Direct eyeball injury

This may be lacerating, blunt or chemical.

Lacerations are easily recognised. It is vital to avoid anything that might raise the intra-ocular pressure and hence empty the eye of its contents.

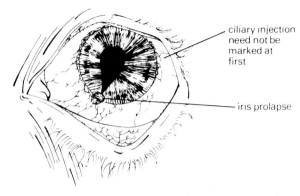

ciliary injection
need not be
marked at
first

iris prolapse

Fig. 14.1 Rupture of the cornea. Intra-occular structures on the outside may mean something alien on the inside.

As far as blunt injury is concerned, the imagination can supply all likely agents, but ball games and fisticuffs must rank high on the list. The front of the eye may fill with blood—a hyphaema—which is recognised when the turbidity has settled by a fluid level (Fig. 14.2).

A blow sufficient to cause such a haemorrhage may well have caused a silent rupture of the globe as well. Blood filling the entire anterior chamber can block the drainage angle and cause an acute secondary glaucoma. If it is not cleaned out soon, it may cause chronic staining of the cornea.

Later developments from blunt trauma may show in after years. Chronic secondary glaucoma can follow fibrosis of the drainage

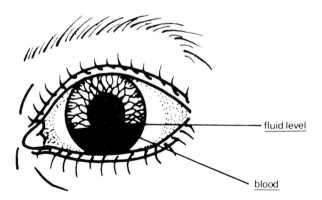

fluid level

blood

Fig. 14.2 Hyphaema. A blow sufficient to cause this may cause other things as well (see Fig. 14.3).

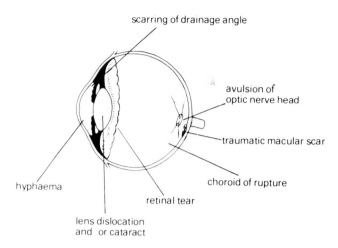

scarring of drainage angle

avulsion of
optic nerve head

traumatic macular scar

choroid of rupture

hyphaema

retinal tear

lens dislocation
and or cataract

Fig. 14.3 Trauma can produce one, or a blend of all of these conditions, not always immediately.

angle, or retinal tears sustained from the original blow can bring about a detachment of the retina at any time—sometimes it happens so long after that the connection may not be suspected.

A lens that has survived traumatic dislocation may not survive traumatic cataract formation (Fig. 14.3).

Chemical injury has a bewildering range, but strong acids or alkalis are particularly popular with bank raiders and have always been familiar on the industrial scene.

Instant washing out with water must be the first move, with the emphasis on instant (Fig. 17.1).

Both chemicals can cause lethal damage. They will distort the eyelids, causing them to adhere to the eye: they can turn in the lashes, opacify the cornea and scarify the drainage angle.

Eyelid injury

There are two situations demanding special attention within 24 hours:
1. laceration involving the lid margin
2. laceration involving the lower canaliculus (Fig. 14.4).

Unless the lid margins are accurately apposed, a notch at the injury site can result in permanent intractable watering, not to mention what exposure or ingrowing lashes can do to the corneal epithelium.

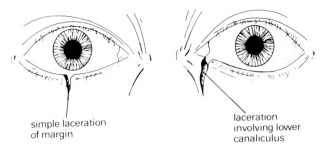

simple laceration
of margin

laceration
involving lower
canaliculus

Fig. 14.4 Laceration of the lid margins. Top priority is restoration of the alliance of the anterior segment and of preserving a channel of communication along the canaliculus.

The watering that follows neglected canalicular injuries is even more distressing—the more so since early surgery might have cured the condition which later surgery almost never can.

Orbital injury

A blow out fracture of the orbital floor is a popular weekend injury, often sustained when the victim's subjective awareness is not at its best (Fig. 14.5). A savage blow forces the orbital contents into the maxillary sinus, where the eye muscles will be trapped by the bony fragments. The tethered eye will not move either upwards or downwards, and if the condition is neglected, never will. It should also be remembered that damage severe enough to smash the bone may

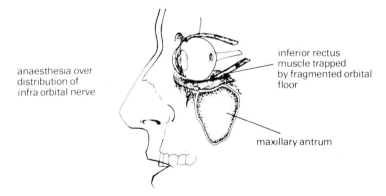

anaesthesia over
distribution of
infra orbital nerve

inferior rectus
muscle trapped
by fragmented orbital
floor

maxillary antrum

Fig. 14.5 Blow out fracture of the orbital floor. Trauma sufficient to smash the bones may do something similar to the eye.

have smashed the eye as well. If the swollen lids have to be forced
open to permit a glimpse of the eye, a comparison with its fellow
for corneal clarity and anterior chamber equality may set the mind
at rest, at least in the short term.

Radiographic examination will confirm or refute any clinical
impression.

It is necessary to elevate the contents of the orbit and keep them
in position with a plate of silicone rubber to make good the defect
in the orbital floor.

Sympathetic ophthalmitis

A penetrating eye injury can give rise to many troubles, but this
condition is perhaps its most fearful complication. In the first two
weeks after an injury, especially one involving the lens and ciliary
body, circulating antibodies to normal eye tissue may be formed.
These antibodies, failing to recognise the eyes as 'self', may then
attack both of them, and they in turn will respond with a smouldering, destructive, inflammatory process.

In practice, it can be assumed that there is no danger during the
first two weeks when the damaged eye should be settling from the
trauma and from the restorative surgery. If it continues to settle,
all is well. However, should the eye flare up again, then the
renewed pain, watering and redness must warn the doctor to
consider enucleation.

Fifteen
Removal of the eye

Many disorders require enucleation of the eye, including over-whelming infection, severe trauma, sympathetic ophthalmitis, painful eye and tumours.

Retinoblastoma

This growth is fortunately as rare as it is malignant, occurring once in rather more than twenty thousand live births.

From its favourite site of origin in the posterior retina, it rapidly fills the vitreous with tumour seedlings. These deposits whiten the normally black pupil, and it is this feature rather than visual loss which catches parental notice.

Most cases present before the age of three, and there is a one in three chance that both eyes may be affected.

Treatment

Enucleation is obligatory for large tumours, but smaller ones may be attacked by a combination of radiotherapy and chemotherapy, both methods curing a large percentage of these unfortunate youngsters.

In known families the hereditary gene appears to be an autosomal dominant with 80 per cent penetrance. This means that half the children will carry the trait, and of this half four out of five will suffer the disease.

Where there is no family history it seems, however, that most cases are sporadic. More and more of these children survive to become parents themselves, and their offspring do not seem to demonstrate any dominant hereditary pattern.

Enucleation

This procedure is not undertaken lightly, and the patient needs lots of support and reassurance. When the patient is a child the parents also need support and reassurance. In some disorders enucleation may be seen as a let down to the patient or the parents hoping for a recovery. In some circumstances, however, enucleation is essential and must be carried out with a minimum of delay. In these circumstances the surgical team must be prepared to help the patient adjust to the loss of an eye in the post-operative period. The pre-operative nursing care before enucleation is routine.

Post-operative care

On completion of the operation the surgeon may either pack the socket or simply apply a pad and bandage; occasionally a shell may be fitted at time of the operation. Much depends on the circumstances, e.g. the amount of swelling present.

The dressing is redone daily and observed for bleeding or discharge. As soon as possible a shell is fitted to keep the socket open in preparation for the fitting of the prothesis in 4 to 6 weeks.

Patients can be up and about as soon as they feel able and are usually ready for discharge in 5–7 days. Instruction is given regarding dressing and follow-up. Sympathy and understanding of their sudden loss are essential if patients are to make a good adjustment.

Sixteen
Drugs commonly used in eye disorders

There are not very many drugs used in the treatment of eye disorders. Some are rarely used whilst a few are very frequently used. Tables 16.1, 16.2, 16.3, 16.4 and 16.5 list some of the more commonly used topical preparations.

Several drugs are given either orally or by injection for the treatment of eye disorders. One commonly used drug is acetazolamide. This drug inhibits carbonic anhydrase, hence reducing the bicarbonate in the aqueous humour and so the amount of water with it. This results in a decrease in the flow of aqueous humour, thus reducing intra-ocular pressure. The normal dose range is up to 1 g per day in divided doses. A slow-release capsule is also available. The drug can be given intravenously. It should only be reconstituted with water immediately before use.

Some patients experience flushing, thirst, headache, drowsiness, dizziness, parasthesia, ataxia and hyperventilation when the drug is first used. Nausea and vomiting may also occur. In the longer term it may produce an abnormality in blood biochemistry known as acidosis which can be potentially dangerous. Changes in respiratory function, e.g. deep irregular breathing, or central nervous system changes, e.g. drowsiness, should be brought to the doctor's attention. As the drug is related to the sulphonamide group, similar side-effects can also occur such as stone formation in the renal tract.

Another drug, dichlorphenamide, has a similar but more prolonged action. It has the same range of side effects, especially in the elderly, such as parasthesia, lack of appetite and depression. Careful observation for changes in mood, etc. should be made and, if noted, reported to the doctor.

In emergency situations when there is a need to reduce intra-ocular pressure, intravenous mannitol or glycerol by mouth is often prescribed. Both these agents are powerful osmotic diuretics. Urinary output should be monitored carefully; the nurse should

Table 16.1 Mydriatics and cycloplegics

Trade name	Approved name	Presentation	Dose range	Indications
Minims atropine S.N.P.	Atropine sulphate 1%	Single dose eye drops	1 drop as required	Pre- and post-operative use. Keratitis, iritis, cyclitis.
Minims cyclopentolate S.N.P.	Cyclopentolate hydrochloride 0.5% and 1%	Single dose eye drops	1 or more drops as required	Mydriatic or cycloplegic for ophthalmic examination.
Minims hyoscine S.N.P.	Hyoscine hydrobromide 0.2%	Single dose eye drops	1 or more drops as required	Rapid onset, short acting, mydriatic and cycloplegic.
Minims tropicamide S.N.P.	Tropicamide 0.5% and 1%	Single dose eye drops	2 drops at 5 min intervals then 1–2 drops 30 min later if required	Mydriatic and cycloplegic.
Minims homatropine S.N.P.	Homatropine hydrobromide 2%	Single dose eye drops	1 or more drops as required	Rapid onset less mydriatic effect than atropine.

Table 16.2 Non-steroid preparations acting on the eye

Trade name	Approved name	Presentation	Dose range	Indications
Vira A	Vidarabine 3%	Ointment	1 cm into conjunctival sac 5 times/day at least, continue for 7 days after healing	Herpes keratoconjunctivitis
Minims neomycin S.N.P.	Neomycin sulp. 0.5%	Single dose eye drops	1–2 drops 5 times/day	Ocular bacterial infections
Albucid	Sulphacetamide sod. 10%, 20%, 30%	Drops	4 drops 2–6 hourly	Ocular infections
Genticin	Gentamicin sulph. 0.3%	Drops	3 or 4 times daily	Ocular bacterial infections
Chloromycetin	Chloramphenicol 1%	Ointment/drops	1 application of ointment or 2 drops 3 hourly or more frequently	Bacterial conjunctivitis
Soframycin	Framycetin sulph. 0.5%	Drops	2 drops 3–4 times daily	Conjunctivitis, blepharitis, styes
Dendrid	Idoxiuridine 0.1%	Drops	Hourly during day 2 hourly during night	Ocular herpes simplex
Zovirax	Acylovir 3%	Ointment	1 cm into conjunctival sac every 4 hours maintain × 3 day post healing	Herpes simplex, keratitis

Table 16.3 Drugs used in treatment of glaucoma

Trade name	Approved name	Presentation	Dose range	Indications
Daranide	Dichlorphenamide	Tablets 50 mg	2–4 tablets initially, 2 tablets 12 hourly	Adjunct in glaucoma
Diamox sustets	Acetazolamide	Capsules 500 mg	1 tablet night and morning (also available in parenteral form)	Adjunct in glaucoma
Eppy S.N.P.	Adrenaline 1 %	Drops	1 drop once or twice daily	Primary open angle and secondary glaucoma
Minims phenylephrine S.N.P.	Phenylephrine 10%	Single dose eye drops	1 drop as required	Temporary covering of intraocular pressure in glaucoma
Minims pilocarpine S.N.P.	Pilocarpine nitrate 1%. 2% and 4%	Single dose eye drops	1 drop 4–6 times daily	Chronic non-congenstive glaucoma and to reverse mydriatics
Timoptol M.S.D.	Timolol (as Maleate 0.25% and 0.5%)	Metered dose eye drops	Initially 1 drop 0.25% soln. changing to 0.5% if required	Ocular hypertension

Table 16.4 Steroid preparations acting on the eye

Trade name	Approved name	Presentation	Dose range	Indications
Vista-methasone N	Betamethasone sod. sulphate 0.1% Neomycin sulphate 0.5%	Drops	1–2 drops hourly	Infected, inflammatory conditions of the ear, eye or nose
Betnesol	Betamethasone sod. phos. 0.1%	Drops, ointment	1 or 2 drops or 1 cm ointment one or two hourly	Non-infected, inflamatory conditions
Chloromycetin 1%	Chloramphenicol 1% Hydrocortisone acetate 0.5%	Ointment	One hourly to once daily depending on severity	Inflammatory ocular infection
Framycort	Framycetin sulph. 0.5% Hydrocortisone acetate 0.5%		2 or 3 times daily	Superficial bacterial ocular infection, conjunctivitis, blepharitis, marginal corneal ulceration
Maxitrol	Dexamethasone 0.1% Neomycin sulph. 0.35% Hypromellose 0.5% Polymixin B sulph. 6000 i.u./ml	Drops	2 drops4–6 times daily	Infected ocular inflammation
Neo-cortef	Hydrocortisone acetate 1.5% Neomycin sulph. 0.5%	Drops	2 drops three or more times daily	Infected ocular inflammation
Minims prednisolone S.N.P.	Prednisolone sod. phos. 0.5%	Drops	1–2 drops as required	Non-infected inflammatory conditions

Table 16.5 Local anaesthetics diagnostics diagnostic agents and artificial tears

Trade name	Approved name	Presentation	Dose range	Indications
Isopto alkaline alcon	Hypromellose 1%	Drops	1 or 2 drops three times daily	Ocular lubrication
Liquefilm tears allergen	Polyvinyl alcohol 1.4%	Drops	1 drop as required	Ocular lubrication
Minims amethocaine S.N.P.	Amethocaine hydrochlor 0.5% and 1%	Single dose eye drops	One or more drops as required	Anaesthesia of the cornea and conjunctiva prior to opthalmic procedures
Minims benoxinate S.N.P.	Oxybuprocaine hydrochloride 0.4%	Single dose eye drops	1 or more drops as required	Anaesthesia of the cornea and conjunctiva prior to ophthalmic procedures
Minims fluorescein S.N.P.	Fluorescein sodium 1%, 2%	Single dose eye drops	1 or more drops as required	Diagnostic stain for ophthalmic procedures
Minims saline S.N.P.	Sodium chloride 0.9%	Single dose eye drops	Use as required	Irrigation of the eye

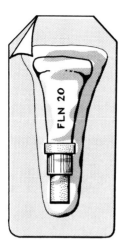

Fig. 16.1 Single application pack.

particularly look out for any retention of urine, especially in the elderly male who may also have a degree of prostatism.

Great care must be taken to prevent the spread of infection when eye drops are instilled.

Many disorders leave the eye vulnerable to bacterial and other infections. Many eye preparations are prescribed in the form of single eye drops in an attempt to limit infection spreading from one patient to another. When multidose containers are used they should be reserved strictly for the patient for whom they were prescribed. Often this also means keeping separate bottles for each eye. Hands should be washed before and after the instillation of the drops or ointment. Patients who are to instill their own drops must also be instructed to wash their hands before and after. Drops must never be transferred from one container to another. Bottles must never be topped up as bacteria introduced can lead to gross contamination. Patients should be informed of how to store and maintain their medication. Many drugs used have a short shelf life and must be discarded once the expiry date is past. Figure 16.1 shows an intact single drop pack whilst Figure 16.2 shows the sequence of opening the pack in preparation for drug administration.

Instillation of eye drops/ointment

There are three methods of instilling eye drops. Firstly, the drop may be placed in the lower conjunctival sac (Fig. 16.3). Secondly,

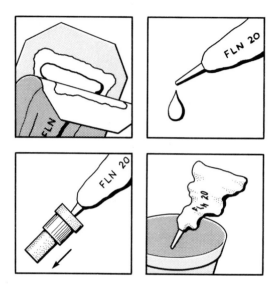

Fig. 16.2 Method of using single application packs.

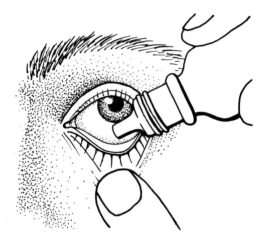

Fig. 16.3 Installation of drops into the lower conjunctival sac.

the drop may be placed over the superior scleral area. The drug thereby flows down over the cornea and pupil (Fig. 16.4). A third technique in a crying infant is to place the drop in the nasal canthus area. The lid is then pulled down so that the drop runs into the conjunctival sac. The main purposes for which eye drops are used are to reduce inflammation, anaesthetise the cornea, dilate or

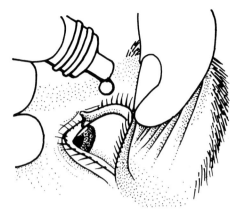

Fig. 16.4 Installation of drops over the superior scleral area.

constrict the pupil, highlight corneal abrasions and lubricate the conjunctiva. The frequency of application very often depends on which effect the drug is expected to have and on the severity of the condition. Some drugs are presented as ointments and are especially useful for night-time application. Before instilling the drops/ointment any secretion should be wiped from the eye and lashes with sterile normal saline swabs (Figs.16.5 and 16.6). The ointment is squeezed from the tube (about a cm) and deposited in the conjunctival sac. Great care must be taken not to contaminate the tube by touching the eye or conjunctiva. Following the application the patient should gently close his eye but must avoid squeezing it tight. This is

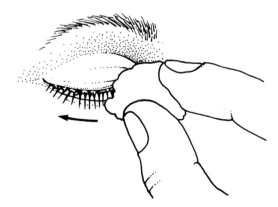

Fig. 16.5 Secretions can be removed by wiping from the inner canthus outwards.

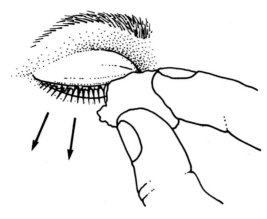

Fig. 16.6 Mucus crusting can be removed by gently stroking downwards.

especially important post-operatively as it raises the intra-ocular pressure and puts a strain on the suture line. Ointments like drops are strictly reserved for the patients for whom they have been supplied. An added precaution which is essential in limiting the spread of eye infection is the isolation of the patient who is infected so that he does not come in contact with patients who require surgery. Isolation and barrier nursing techniques are described in all good foundation nursing textbooks and will not be elaborated on here.

Seventeen
Common nursing procedures

Eye compresses

There are many reasons for applying compresses, which may be either warm or cold depending on the pathology. Compresses are an aid to cleansing; they decrease pain, help to reduce ecchymosis and/or oedema and reduce inflammation. Warm compresses increase the blood supply to a local area, while cold compresses constrict or decrease the blood supply. The compress is usually applied for up to 20 minutes at a time, four or more times daily. When commercially prepared compresses are used, the patient is best placed in the supine position so that the compress stays in position more easily. Warm compresses are covered with a sterile towel to maintain their warmth, whilst cold compresses are left exposed, to maintain a cold temperature.

A long established method of applying heat to the eye is hot spoon bathing. Suitable really only for adults, a well padded wooden spoon is soaked in hot water and then held in close proximity to the eye. It must not touch the eye; the heat radiates from the pad and steam evaporates from it. The steam loosens secretions and helps to clean the eye, whilst the heat helps to reduce inflammation, eases pain and is generally soothing. As the patient usually performs the procedure himself he is actively involved and this helps to boost confidence and adds to the efficiency of the process.

Irrigation of the eye

This is a very simple procedure and can on occasion prevent blindness or at very least limit damage. The most common use is to remove strong irritating chemicals from the eye. The longer the chemical is in contact with the eye the more serious is the damage caused, hence immediate irrigation is essential. The eye is washed out copiously using plain tap water. This also dilutes the chemical

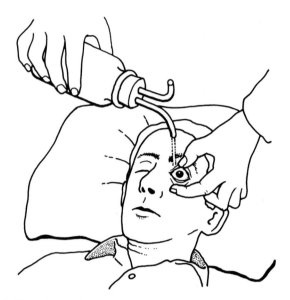

Fig. 17.1 Technique of irrigating an eye.

and so reduces the amount of damage. The patient (casualty) should
be lying down head positioned to one side (Fig. 17.1). The eyelids
are held open by firmly holding the upper lid against the superior
orbital rim with the index or middle finger, while the lower lid is
pulled down with the thumb. The water should then be poured into
the conjunctival sac and allowed to run over the cornea.

Eighteen
Nursing care of the visually handicapped

Before reading this chapter through, try a little experiment. Go into a familiar room and stand in the centre. Close your eyes and then turn round through 360° once or twice; now, still keeping your eyes closed try to locate the door you entered the room by. The chances are you will have very great difficulty in locating the door and more than likely knock into the furniture. Do not try this experiment in a room in which you might injure yourself. Of course, when you can't find the door you can open your eyes and reorientate yourself: but what of the person who is blind? The blind person finds himself in this position every time he enters a strange room. At home he can find his way around because he has become familiar with its layout. The blind person memorises exactly where everything is and they by keeping everything in its allotted place he can find things relatively easily. The person born blind can readily master the layout of a new environment and some move around with such ease it is difficult to appreciate that they are blind. The person who has just lost his sight has much greater difficulty in moving around safely. It is normal practice to orientate patients to the ward layout when they are admitted. They are shown which part of the ward their bed is in, the position of toilets, dayroom, outside telephone, sister's office and so on. Note the use of the word 'shown'. The blind person or those whose vision is very poor require to be orientated in a different way. Coming into hospital is in itself stressful for most people, being blind makes it even more so. The person who has recently become blind can easily create an image of the room or ward if it is described to him. Start with the approximate size of the room, and then go on to the position of the bed and other furniture. Lead the person round the room allowing him to touch the walls and furniture. By doing this the dimensions and layout will soon become familiar. Do not teach too much at any one time—initially, just enough should be shown to the patient to make him feel secure. Allow the patient to unpack his own case and to position dressing-gown, slippers and other personal items in his locker. Nurses often go round moving things about and tidying up. Moving things makes it impossible for the patient to find things without unnecessary groping around. Make sure that the patient can locate the nurse call bell and ask him to ring if he requires anything. Reassure him that there will always be someone quite close by and that you will orientate him to the other parts of the ward later, when he has got used to being in the ward for a few hours.

Whilst there are no hard and fast rules for communicating and caring for the visually handicapped the following points should be used as a guide.

Communication. The blind person is at a serious disadvantage in so far that he is unable to identify who is addressing him. When speaking, always address the person by name and let him know who you are and what your position is. Failure to do this may mean that the person does not know whether it is he who is being spoken to or not. Also, if you do not know his name touch him on the arm before speaking.

Always state your business clearly so that he knows what is going on around him. For example, if you have come to straighten his bed tell him this is what you are about to do. The same applies if you are giving him a cup of tea. Do not leave tea on the locker or bed table without saying it is there. Do not assume that he has heard you place it there. When giving lunch take a few moments to let him know what is for lunch and how it is arranged on the plate relative to him: relate the position of the food on the plate to the face of a clock; for example, the meat is at six-o-clock, the potatoes at three and so on. Meat and vegetables should be cut up into manageable positions; do not mince or liquidise unless for other medical/nursing reasons: minced-up food has a uniform taste and texture and is not as appetising.

At the end of any procedure or conversation tell the patient you are leaving, making sure he understands this and that he can call if he wishes anything further. If you do not do this he may well find himself in the embarrasing situation of talking to air. Also remember to introduce him to neighbouring patients as he may not know they are close by and so deny himself the opportunity of a friendly chat. Before leaving, make sure you have replaced everything the same as before so that the patient can find things easily and does not have to grope around, possibly knocking things over. If an item has to be moved tell the patient and show him its new position.

Activity. The visually handicapped person requires exercise like anyone else, only he may experience difficulty in taking adequate exercise for fear of injuring himself or causing other damage. When walking with a blind person, allow him to take your arm and walk half a pace ahead of him. Let him follow you rather than push him along in front of you. Keep up a reasonable commentary about the environment and any obstacles, whether there are steps and if so are they up or down. There is no need to walk very slowly, except for good medical reasons, so that normal walking pace should be encouraged. If other activity is needed and desirable, a safe place in the ward or physiotherapy department can be made available and appropriate exercises allowed. This would include stretching, extension and flexion exercises and a range of motion activities to get limbs and joints moving. Small weights can be held in the hands, or rowing machines, static bicycles, wall-bar exercises and so on can all be performed quite safely by the visually handicapped.

When showing the blind person to a chair put his hand on the back of the chair and allow him to sit down on his own. There is no need to physically sit him down! the same on getting up. If he uses a walking aid, place this in an appropriate position and let him get up on his own. If you are to guide him, simply allow him to stand and take your arm as mentioned above.

A common problem the visually handicapped and people with other handicaps experience is being addressed via a third person. Nurses and others will often ask questions of someone accompanying the handicapped person rather than ask him directly. This is most irritating to the handicapped person. Because there is no eye contact may people raise their voices to attract attention; again this is an unnecessary tactic, unless the handicapped person is also hard of hearing.

The blind person is a normal human being who happens to be blind. He dislikes being talked down to as much as any other person. This is especially so in dealing with the person who has recently lost his sight for whatever reason. He has already suffered a severe blow to his self-esteem, and is very often depressed and bewildered. The newly blind person goes through a period of grieving in the same way as someone who is grieving over the loss of a loved one. The blind person needs to be treated with the same respect as any other person. Preservation of his dignity and enhancement of his self-esteem should be a prime aim in nursing care.

Appendix two
Contact lenses

Contact lenses are foreign bodies applied to the cornea in the hope that visual improvement or emotional relief from discarding spectacles will compensate for the insult to the eye of their application. Made from a variety of synthetic transparent materials of differing physical attributes, they are accepted by the eye only in the presence of a normal fluid exchange across the corneal surface and an adequate supply of tears.

These conditions are not always met. Fluid balance throughout the body fluctuates as the normal hormonal cycles fluctuate, and when these cycles are further unbalanced by the contraceptive pill, pregnancy or impending abortion, intolerance of contact lenses may be the first indication. Should the tear secretion decline below a certain critical level, then this intolerance becomes permanent.

Even healthy eyes have their problems. Coarsely fitted lenses depriving the anterior corneal surface of oxygen will cause a hazy oedema of the epithelium. Overwearing of well-fitted lenses will produce the same result, and if carried to foolish lengths, may induce the growth of superficial new vessels around the corneoscleral limbus—presumably to make up the oxygen normally supplied by the tears.

With this baleful array of hazards it is a wonder that people wear contact lenses at all. They do so for a variety of reasons. Vanity and cosmetic satisfaction can lead to a tolerance of the most appalling discomforts, and most contact lenses are worn for these reasons. However, there can be no doubt that eyes with extreme refractive errors see more effectively with such lenses than they do with standard glasses. The visual field enlarges when unhampered by thick spectacle frames, and the distorting periphery of a thick lens is not used when a lens of equivalent strength is placed upon the eye. Central vision also sharpens, because contact with the eye is a much more natural optical arrangement than glasses in a frame. The pity is that it is not a more natural corneal arrangement.

Such lenses have their uses for medical reasons. Unilateral aphakics who have normal vision in the other eye may regain binocular function when a contact lens comes near to restoring the optical balance of the eye to what it was before the cataract was removed.

An abnormal curvature of the cornea (keratoconus) not only induces myopia, but also thin opaque corneal stroma at the summit of the cone. A judiciously designed lens may not only prevent this disaster, but may improve the vision as well and delay the need for corneal grafting. When corneal ulcers refuse to heal, stitching the eyelids together (tarsorrhaphy) is not always acceptable, especially in an only eye. A contact lens can be applied as a bandage to allow the corneal epithelium to regenerate without external disturbance. The lids stay open. The patient may continue to see, and the sceptical will also see that covering the cornea is not just a device to conceal therapeutic defeat.

Contact lens wearers complain from time to time of irritable eyes. This is not surprising as the potential cause has been applied by themselves. Corneal abrasions, erosions, infections and frank assault from trying to remove a contact lens that may not be in position, are all ways in which this may happen. More common still is a grumbling conjunctivitis caused by simple intolerance to the lens material, or allergy to the endless variety of solutions available for them to steep in. The routine examination ritual will show which part of the external eye has been damaged, and most symptoms will clear away when the lens is taken out. Most symptoms will stay away if the lens is kept out, at least until all the signs and any doubts over the suitability of the lens have cleared away as well.

Further reading

General

Birrell J F 1982 Diseases of the nose throat and ear, 9th edn. Wright, Bristol

Chilman A M, Thomas M 1986 Understanding nursing care 3rd edn. Churchill Livingstone, Edinburgh

Hall, I S, Colman B H 1981 Diseases of the nose throat and ear. Churchill Livingstone, Edinburgh

Miles Foxen E H 1980 Lecture notes on diseases of the ear nose and throat, 5th edn. Blackwell Scientific Publications, Oxford.

Pracy R, Seigler J, Stell P M, Rogers J 1981 Ear nose and throat surgery and nursing 1st edn.. Hodder and Stoughton, London

Saunders W H, Havener W H, Keith C F, Havener G 1979 Nursing care in eye ear nose and throat disorders, 4th edn. C V Mosby Company, St Louis

Introduction

Brill E L, Kilts D F 1980 Foundations for nursing, 1st edn. Appleton-Century-Crofts, New York.

Chapter one

Anwar A, Atherton V 1981 Dizziness in the elderly: giddy in old age. Nursing Mirror 159 (9): 35–36

Bozian M W, Clark H M 1980 Counteracting sensory changes in aging. American Journal of Nursing 80 (3): 473–477

Bridges M 1982 Extended cortical mastoidectomy and lympanoplasty for chronic otitis media. Nursing Times 78 (3): 101–107

Brown M 1978 Glue ear. Nursing Mirror 147 (5): 32–33

Fairweather W 1981 Care of adults with hearing loss. Nursing (Oxford) 28: 1236–1238

Gibson W, Kanagaonkar G 1979 Practical nursing: syringing the ear. Nursing Mirror 148 (7): 24–25

Klein D 1983 Hearing impairment of the ear, nose and throat. Nursing (Oxford) 2 (18): 517–518

Levine B 1983 Hearing loss—the invisible disability. Nursing (Oxford) 2 (18): 525–529

Lindsay M 1983 The roaring deafness. Nursing Times Feb: 61–63

Montgomery G 1981 Audiocentric attitudes—a barrier to understanding deaf people. Nursing (Oxford) 28: 1231–1234

Owen-Smith M 1979 Bomb blast injuries. Nursing Mirror 149 (13): 35–39

Ross T 1981 Deafness: breaking through the sound barrier. Nursing Mirror 152 (21): 20–23

Roughneen M J 1983 Ear syringing. Nursing (Oxford) 2 (18): 530–531

Sataloff R T, Colton C M 1981 Otitis media: a common childhood infection. American Journal of Nursing 81 (8): 1480–1483

Stokes D 1981 Deafness. Nursing (Oxford) 28: 1228–1230

Voke J 1979 Sounding out the wares. Nursing Mirror 149 (23): 40–41

Voke J 1979 The ear: on balance, it very important. Nursing Mirror 149 (24): 34–35

Chapter two

Black J M, Arnold P L 1982 Facial fractures. America Journal of Nursing 82 (7): 1086–1088

Brinacombe J 1978 Surgery lets a baby breathe through his nose. Nursing Mirror 147 (22): 43–46

Callery P 1981 Tonsillectomy, adenoidectomy and bilateral myringotomy. Nursing Times 77 (28): 1201–1204

Felstein I 1979 Snoring: the sufferer who doesn't suffer. Nursing Mirror 148 (15): 42–43

Harries M 1983 Epistaxis in the elderly. Nursing (Oxford) 2 (18): 533–535

Honeysett J 1982 Epistaxis. Nursing Times 78 (14): 578–581

Pritchard B J 1983 Craniofacial resection. Nursing (Oxford) 2 (18): 536–537

Chapter three

Baines A 1979 Keeping up good appearances. Nursing Mirror 149 (10):38

Bersani G, William C 1983 Oral care for cancer patients. American Journal of Nursing 83 (4): 533–536

Cundey B 1981 Artificial teeth: a bit of a mouthful. Nursing Mirror 152 (15): 30–31

Frank A S T 1973 The mouth in old age. Nursing Times 1292–1293

Gibson I M 1983 Tracheostomy management. Nursing (Oxford) 2 (18): 532–533

Honeysett J 1981 Swimming aids for laryngectomees. Nursing Times 77 (24): 1045–1046

Howarth H 1977 Mouth care procedures for the very ill. Nursing Times 73 (10): 354–355

Keddie G M 1981 Total laryngectomy for advanced carcinoma of the larynx. Nursing Times 77 (27): 1155–1157

Knowles M H 1983 Infections of the ear nose and throat. Nursing (Oxford) 2 (18): 515–516

Larsen G L 1982 Rehabilitation for the patient with head and neck cancer. American Journal of Nursing 82 (1): 119–120

McCormick G P et al 1982 Artificial speech devices. American Journal of Nursing 82 (1): 121–122

Nally F F 1977 Infections of the mouth. Nursing Times 73 (37): 1275–1278

Reeves J 1981 Speak in support. Nursing Mirror 152 (4): 32–33

Schweiger J L, Schweiger J W, Lang J W 1980 Oral assessment: How to do it. American Journal of Nursing 80 (4): 654–657

Serra A M 1983 Lasers in ENT. Nursing (Oxford) 2 (18): 532–533

Smith C J 1976 Oral leukoplakia. Nursing Times 771–772

Stokes D, Jones A W 1983 Laryngectomy—nursing care and a patient's view. Nursing (Oxford) 2 (18): 520–521

Appendix one

D.H.S.S. 1979 General guidance for hearing aid users. D.H.S.S., Edinburgh

Harford E R 1979 Guidelines for hearing problems: substituting management for myth. Geriatrics 34 (12): 69–72

Chapter four

Norman S 1982 The pupil check. The American Journal of Nursing 82 (4): 588–591

O'Callaghan B 1983 Structure and function of the eye. Nursing (Oxford) 2 (17): 487–489

Voke J 1982 Vision, queen of the senses 1—Optics of the eye. Nursing Times 78 (35): 1463–1466

Voke J 1982 Vision 2—How the eye regulates light entry. Nursing
    Times 78 (36): 1506–1507
Voke J 1982 Vision 3—How the pressure is maintained and the
    consequences of glaucoma. Nursing Times 78 (31): 1557–1560
Voke J 1982 Vision 4—Chemical in the retina which initiate vision.
    Nursing Time 78 (38): 1599–1600
Voke J 1981 Vision: seeing is believing. Nursing Mirror 153 (4): 37–39

Chapter five

Wolfsberger J 1981 Precious eyesight. Nursing Times 77 (4): 158–161

Chapter seven

Gallagher M A 1981 Corneal transplantation. The American Journal of
    Nursing 81 (10): 1845 (Oct 1981)
Haves M J, Ellis P P 1983 Tearing in the geriatric patient: causes and
    treatments, Geriatrics 38 (3): 113–118
Jeffree C 1984 Dacryocystorhinostomy 80 (3): 35–37
Treharne J D 1976 Trachoma. Nursing Times 72 (14): 523–525

Chapter eight

Wright M J 1983 The red eye. Nursing (Oxford) 2 (17): 503–505

Chapter nine

Cook J 1981 Cataract extraction under local anaesthetic. Nursing Times
    77 (21): 894–895
Ingram R M, Banerjee D, Traynar M J, Thompson R K 1983 Day case
    cataract surgery. British Journal of Ophthalmology 67 (5): 278–281
Kidger J 1983 Cataracts. Nursing (Oxford) 2 (17): 511–512
Woodward E G, Morris J A 1982 Contact lenses in aphakic children.
    Nursing Times 78 (17): 725–726

Chapter ten

Ghafour I M, Allan D, Foulds W S 1983 Common causes of blindness
    and visual handicap in the West of Scotland. British Journal of
    Ophthalmology 67 (4): 209–213
McKean J M, Elkington A R 1983 Compliances with treatment of
    patients with chronic open angle glaucoma. British Journal of
    Ophthalmology 67 (1): 46–49

Resler M M, Tumulty G 1983 Glaucoma update. The American Journal of Nursing 83 (5): 752–756 (May 1983)
Travers J P 1978 Primary open angle glaucoma. Nursing Times 74 (3): 103–104

Chapter eleven

Timms C 1983 Squint. Nursing (Oxford) 2 (17): 495–496

Chapter twelve

Smith J S 1983 Ophthalmic problems in general nursing. Nursing (Oxford) 2 (17): 507–508

Chapter thirteen

Graham J M 1982 Vitrectomy surgery. Nursing Times 78 (50): 2113–2117
Ingram R M, Banerjee D, Traynor M J, Thompson R K 1983 Day case cataract surgery. British Journal of Ophthalmology 67: 278–281
Macfadyen J S 1980 Caring for the patient with a primary retinal detachment. The American Journal of Nursing 80 (5): 920–921

Chapter fourteen

Bowman K 1983 Blindness following a fall at work. Nursing Times 79 (32): 53–54
Cullen J F 1983 Eye injuries. Hospital update 10 (9): 1103–1114
Fletcher D 1981 Intra-occular foreign bodies: an eye for treatment. Nursing Mirror 152 (17): 35–36
Lowe J 1983 Nursing management of eye injuries. Nursing (Oxford) 2 (17): 490–495
Seewoodhary M 1983 Common presentations in accident and emergency nursing (Oxford) 2 (17): 498–501

Chpater sixteen

Wong D L, Dornan C R 1982 Nursing care in childhood cancer: retinoblastoma. The American Journal of Nursing 82 (3): 425–431

Chapter seventeen

Farquharson H R L 1983 Blindness. Nursing (Oxford) 2 (17): 511–512

Appendix two

Josse E 1984 Corneal abscess from soft contact lens. Nursing Times 26 (12): Supplement 3–4

Ruben M 1976 The pros and cons of soft contact lens. Nursing Times 72 (26): 1018–1020

Index